D0764313

The Hippocampus in Clinical Neuroscience

Frontiers of Neurology and Neuroscience

Vol. 34

Series Editor

J. Bogousslavsky Montreux

The Hippocampus in Clinical Neuroscience

Volume Editors

K. Szabo Mannheim
M.G. Hennerici Mannheim

31 figures, 13 in color, and 5 tables, 2014

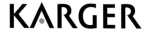

Basel · Freiburg · Paris · London · New York · Chennai · New Delhi ·
Bangkok · Beijing · Shanghai · Tokyo · Kuala Lumpur · Singapore · Sydney

Frontiers of Neurology and Neuroscience

Vols. 1–18 were published as Monographs in Clinical Neuroscience

Prof. Dr. Kristina Szabo
Prof. Dr. Michael G. Hennerici
Department of Neurology
UniversitätsMedizin Mannheim
Theodor-Kutzer-Ufer 1-3
DE–68167 Mannheim (Germany)

Library of Congress Cataloging-in-Publication Data

The hippocampus in clinical neuroscience / volume editors, K. Szabo, M.G. Hennerici.
   p. ; cm. -- (Frontiers of neurology and neuroscience, ISSN 1660-4431
; vol. 34)
   Includes bibliographical references and indexes.
   ISBN 978-3-318-02567-5 (hard cover : alk. paper) -- ISBN 978-3-318-02568-2
(e-ISBN)
   I. Szabo, Kristina, editor. II. Hennerici, M. (Michael), editor. III.
Series: Frontiers of neurology and neuroscience ; v. 34. 1660-4431
   [DNLM: 1. Hippocampus. W1 MO568C v. 34 2014 / WL 314]
   QP383.25
   612.8'25--dc23
                                                                2014010411

Bibliographic Indices. This publication is listed in bibliographic services, including Current Contents® and Index Medicus.

© Copyright 2014 by S. Karger AG, P.O. Box, CH–4009 Basel (Switzerland)
www.karger.com
Printed in Germany on acid-free and non-aging paper (ISO 9706) by Kraft Druck, Ettlingen
ISSN 1660–4431
e-ISSN 1662–2804
ISBN 978–3–318–02567–5
e-ISBN 978–3–318–02568–2

Contents

List of Contributors

Dr. Pamela Banta Lavenex
Laboratory for Experimental Research on
Behavior, Institute of Psychology
University of Lausanne, Géopolis 4524
CH–1015 Lausanne (Switzerland)
E-Mail pamela.bantalavenex@unil.ch

Dr. Dennis Chan
Herchel Smith Building for Brain and
Mind Sciences
University of Cambridge
Forvie Site, Robinson Way
Cambridge CB2 0SZ (UK)
E-Mail dc598@medschl.cam.ac.uk

Dr. Anastasios Chatzikonstantinou
Department of Neurology
UniversitätsMedizin Mannheim
Theodor-Kutzer-Ufer 1-3
DE–68167 Mannheim (Germany)
E-Mail chatziko@neuro.ma.uni-heidelberg.de

Prof. Dr. Andreas Draguhn
Institut für Physiologie und Pathophysiologie,
Universität Heidelberg
Im Neuenheimer Feld 326
DE–69120 Heidelberg (Germany)
E-Mail andreas.draguhn@
          physiologie.uni-heidelberg.de

Dr. rer. nat. Maren Engelhardt
Institute of Neuroanatomy
Center for Biomedicine and Medical Technology
Mannheim (CBTM)
Medical Faculty Mannheim/Heidelberg
University
Ludolf-Krehl Str. 13-17
DE–68167 Mannheim (Germany)
E-Mail maren.engelhardt@
          medma.uni-heidelberg.de

Dr. Grégoire Favre
Unité de Psychiatrie et de Psychothérapie
Département de Médecine
Université de Fribourg
Chemin du Musée 5
CH–1700 Fribourg (Switzerland)
E-Mail gregoire.favre@unifr.ch

Dr. Alex Förster
Department of Neurology
UniversitätsMedizin Mannheim
Theodor-Kutzer-Ufer 1-3
DE–68167 Mannheim (Germany)
E-Mail alex.foerster@umm.de

Dr. Achim Gass
Department of Neurology
UniversitätsMedizin Mannheim
Theodor-Kutzer-Ufer 1-3
DE–68167 Mannheim (Germany)
E-Mail achim.gass@medma.uni-heidelberg.de

Prof. Dr. Michael G. Hennerici
Department of Neurology
UniversitätsMedizin Mannheim
Theodor-Kutzer-Ufer 1-3
DE–68167 Mannheim (Germany)
E-Mail hennerici@neuro.ma.uni-heidelberg.de

Martin Keller
Institut für Physiologie und Pathophysiologie
Universität Heidelberg
Im Neuenheimer Feld 326
DE–69120 Heidelberg (Germany)
E-Mail martin.k.keller@gmail.com

Prof. Dr. Pierre Lavenex
Laboratory for Experimental Research on
Behavior, Institute of Psychology
University of Lausanne, Géopolis 4343
CH–1015 Lausanne (Switzerland)
E-Mail pierre.lavenex@unil.ch

Dr. K.K. Moodley
Clinical Research Fellow
Clinical Imaging Sciences Centre
Brighton and Sussex Medical School
Falmer, Brighton BN1 9RR (UK)
E-Mail K.moodley2@bsms.ac.uk

Frauke Nees, PhD
Department of Cognitive and Clinical
Neuroscience, Central Institute of Mental Health
Square J 5
DE–68159 Mannheim (Germany)
E-Mail frauke.nees@zi-mannheim.de

Prof. Dr. Bertram Opitz
School of Psychology, University of Surrey
Guildford GU2 7XH (UK)
E-Mail b.opitz@surrey.ac.uk

Dr. Sebastian Pohlack
Department of Cognitive and
Clinical Neuroscience
Central Institute of Mental Health, Square J 5
DE–68159 Mannheim (Germany)
E-Mail sebastian.pohlack@zi-mannheim.de

Dr. Susanne Reichinnek
Institut für Physiologie und Pathophysiologie
Universität Heidelberg
Im Neuenheimer Feld 326
DE–69120 Heidelberg (Germany)
E-Mail susanne.reichinnek@gmx.de

Prof. Dr. med. Christian Schultz
Institute of Neuroanatomy
Center for Biomedicine and Medical Technology
Mannheim (CBTM)
Medical Faculty Mannheim/Heidelberg
University
Ludolf-Krehl Str. 13-17
DE–68167 Mannheim (Germany)
E-Mail christian.schultz@
       medma.uni-heidelberg.de

Frauke Steiger
Department of Cognitive and Clinical
Neuroscience, Central Institute of Mental Health
Square J 5
DE–68159 Mannheim (Germany)
E-Mail frauke.steiger@zi-mannheim.de

Prof. Dr. Kristina Szabo
Department of Neurology
UniversitätsMedizin Mannheim
Theodor-Kutzer-Ufer 1-3
DE–68167 Mannheim (Germany)
E-Mail szabo@neuro.ma.uni-heidelberg.de

Prof. Laurent Tatu
Department of Neuromuscular diseases
CHU Jean-Minjoz
Boulevard Fleming
FR–25030 Besançon Cedex (France)
E-Mail laurent.tatu@univ-fcomte.fr

Dr. Fabrice Vuillier
Departments of Anatomy and Neurology
CHU Besançon
2 Boulevard Fleming
FR–25000 Besançon (France)
E-Mail fabrice.vuillier@univ-fcomte.fr

Manon Wicking
Department of Cognitive and Clinical
Neuroscience, Central Institute of Mental Health
Square J 5
DE–68159 Mannheim (Germany)
E-Mail manon.wicking@zi-mannheim.de

Prof. Dr. Katja Wingenfeld
Department of Psychiatry
Charité University Berlin
Campus Benjamin Franklin
Eschenallee 3
DE–14050 Berlin (Germany)
E-Mail katja.wingenfeld@charite.de

Prof. Dr. Oliver T. Wolf
Department of Cognitive Psychology
Ruhr University Bochum
GAFO 02/386
Universitätsstrasse 150
DE–44780 Bochum (Germany)
E-Mail oliver.t.wolf@rub.de

Preface

This publication is the result of many years of clinical and academic interest in the hippocampus, perhaps the most intriguing structure of the human brain. Damage to this structure, one of the oldest parts of the brain integrated in highly complex networks, causes symptoms ranging from transient dysfunction accompanied by tiny lesions to severely debilitating cognitive disorders with marked tissue loss. Besides the motivation to provide information on clinical function and dysfunction of the hippocampus from a neurologist's point of view, several other chapters arose from discussions with expert colleagues from other neuroscience disciplines participating in our collaborative research effort dedicated to 'learning, memory, and brain plasticity'.

Although overlaps between the different fields of hippocampus research, by their very nature, cannot be avoided completely, the editors allocated the individual contributions to three general sections. Section 1 of the book summarizes the current knowledge regarding structure and physiology of the hippocampus, and establishes the ties to basic neuroscience. Section 2 deals with the function of the hippocampus in humans and its assessment. Finally, Section 3 reviews common pathological conditions affecting the hippocampus with a chapter devoted to the effects of stress on hippocampus-mediated memory function and its relevance for selected disorders.

We wish to thank the editorial staff at Karger Publishers for their continuous guidance and advice, and all of the contributing authors for the time and effort they have invested in this project. We hope the reader will enjoy the book as much as we did preparing it, and will find it instructional and useful.

Michael G. Hennerici, Mannheim
Kristina Szabo, Mannheim

Szabo K, Hennerici MG (eds): The Hippocampus in Clinical Neuroscience.
Front Neurol Neurosci. Basel, Karger, 2014, vol 34, pp 1–5 (DOI: 10.1159/000361068)

Introduction

Michael G. Hennerici

Department of Neurology, UniversitätsMedizin Mannheim, University of Heidelberg, Mannheim, Germany

An impairment of memory is a frequent finding in patients with neurodegenerative diseases such as Parkinson's disease, Alzheimer's disease, and others associated with memory deficits, which are correlated with reduced hippocampal function – both postmortem studies and in vivo brain investigations using modern brain imaging have reported similar results. In addition, transient memory deficits have been documented in diffusion-weighted imaging magnetic resonance investigations, suggesting regional white matter changes as well as microstructural alterations of the neurons at the level of hippocampal formation. High-resolution volumetry and diffusibility studies using more recent technologies aim to investigate macro- and microstructural changes of the hippocampal formation in individuals with early neurodegenerative diseases even without dementia (Parkinson's disease), which is challenging at a preclinical stage.

Carlesimo et al. [1] reported declarative memory impairment in patients that may be predicted by the rate of microstructural alterations in the hippocampal formation as detected by diffusion tensor imaging analysis. Similar findings have been demonstrated in healthy aged individuals and patients with mild cognitive impairment, suggesting that these biomarkers are reasonably better predictors for memory impairment than hippocampal volumetry. The reasons for these results are not entirely known; however, an increase of diffusibility might be an expression of an enlargement of the extracellular space due to altered architecture, resulting from immaturity or degeneration. Direct changes of secondary degeneration due to disruption of white matter tracts connecting other main structures may ultimately lead to cortical dysfunction. This stresses the importance of a complex network not only within the hippocampus, but also outside in both the subcortical and cortical areas. It is therefore of utmost importance to understand and always remember the anatomical and functional correlation of hippocampal abnormalities and deficits in both diseased and healthy ageing.

These fascinating aspects of both function and anatomy as evidenced by modern neuroscience have already been challenged by the ancient anatomists [2]. The elegant curved structure of the hippocampus led ancient scholars to name this formation the 'hippocampus cornu ammonis', the coiled horn of the ram. Ammon's horn reflects hippocampal CA1 structures next to CA2 and CA3. Many functions such as inventiveness, spirit, and even consciousness were proposed by the 16th-century anatomist Giulio Cesare Aranzi, who coined the name because of its similarity to the tropical fish (see Tatu and Vuillier [this vol., p. 20; fig. 2]). Once microscopy became available, the hippocampus formation with its typical neuronal arrangement fascinated former scientists, not at least because of its unique cortical structure. In the 19th century, Camillo Goegi illustrated the unique organization of the hippocampus using his innovative staining procedure (see Schultz and Engelhardt [this vol., p. 9; fig. 1a]).

During the 18th and 19th centuries and even in the early 20th century, the hippocampal formation was considered to be part of the olfactory system, probably because of its impressive size in animals with large olfactory bulbs, such as rodents. In addition, early neurophysiological studies indicated olfactory sensations in patients suffering seizures originated from the hippocampal area [John Hughlings Jackson and Charles Beevor (1890) as well as Wilder Penfield and Theodor Erickson (1941)]. However, Alf Brodal (1947) argued against a major role of the hippocampus in olfactory function. He claimed that fibers arising in the olfactory bulb did not directly connect to hippocampal cellular structures. He also cited studies from other investigators who observed similar cortical structures as the hippocampal formation even in anosmatic and microsmatic animals such as dolphins and whales. As often in biological sciences, concepts related to standard technologies have to be revised once more sensitive techniques become available. Better staining conditions in the late 20th century provided evidence that the entorhinal cortex in rodents receives a massive direct projection from the olfactory bulb. Furthermore, even in the monkey, part of the entorhinal cortex is directly connected to the lateral olfactory tract. Interestingly, olfactory memory tasks in functional imaging studies are often related to the hippocampus.

Another important hypothesis was proposed by James W. Papez (1937), who proposed a circuit that interconnected cortical and subcortical structures, which today bears his name. Like others, he proposed the idea of emotional and behavioral aspects of hippocampal function and might have been supported by Heinrich Klüver, a psychologist, and Paul Bucy, a neurologist (1937). Klüver and Bucy reported the constellation now known as the Klüver-Bucy syndrome, which includes aspects of visually guided behavior and modifications of emotional expression. Again, these speculations were discouraged by studies of several investigators who in the late 20th century showed that loss of fear and other behavioral alterations could be attributed to damage to the amygdala connections with visual projections of the infratemporal cortex.

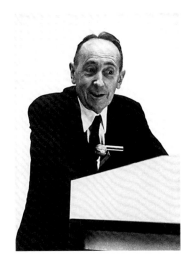

Fig. 1. Richard Jung (1911–1986), private collection.

Richard Jung (fig. 1), a neurologist in Freiburg (Germany), and Alois Kornmüller noted that desynchronization of the neocortical EEG was linked to what they called 'theta-activity' in the rabbit hippocampus. In the 1950s this activity was related to attention, associated and expressed during particular learning conditions. Consistent other findings imply the involvement of the hippocampus to control attention.

By the end of the 19th and beginning of the 20th centuries, neurologists such as Paul Broca, the French psychologist Théodule-Armand Ribot, and the neurosurgeon John Hughlings Jackson reported results from patients with abnormalities of memory according to traumatic, surgical, and ischemic lesions. Observations by Carl Wernicke in 1881 are still well known among medical students because of the Wernicke-Korsakov psychosis bearing his name, a condition that was associated with massive alcohol consumption and simultaneous nutritional deficits, leading to thiamine deficiency treated with high-dose vitamin B substitution. He observed that patients with this illness developed (among other signs and symptoms) typical elements of mental confusion, coma, and eventually death. Postmortem findings were similar to those described by Sergei S. Korsakov and were pathologically associated with lesions in the mammillary bodies, parts of the thalamus, and gray matter structures in the upper brainstem, all heavily connected with the hippocampal network.

Direct evidence for hippocampal involvement in memory came from observations made in famous patients who suffered bilateral surgical removal of substantial parts of the hippocampal formation within the mesial temporal lobes performed because of intractable seizures. The most famous of these, H.M., was an epileptic patient who was left with substantial global amnesia after surgery (anterograde and retrograde amnesia). While he could remember and rehearse brief episodes without distraction, he completely failed during stress and after short intervals. It only became a general concept during the last decades of the 20th century that more than one type of memory

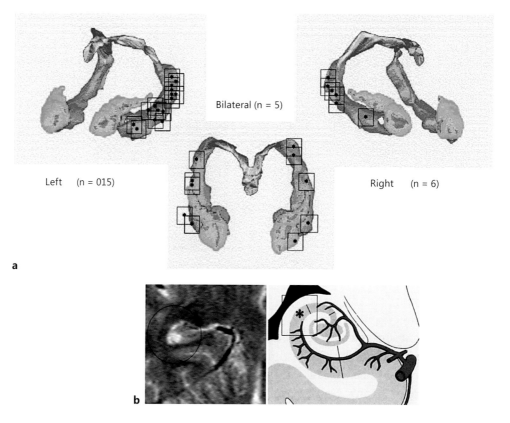

Bilateral (n = 5)

Left   (n = 015)

Right   (n = 6)

a

b

Fig. 2. a Schematic drawing of focal diffusion-weighted imaging lesions located in 26 patients with transient global amnesia and in a segmented hippocampus (projection in neurologic convention: left side = left hemisphere). **b** T2 lesion and the related neurovascular anatomy of the hippocampal structures. Schematic drawing of the borderzone between the upper and lower hippocampal artery: the hypoxia-susceptible sector of Sommer. From [4], reprinted with permission.

and only one of which involved the hippocampus were actually to be separated: episodic memory versus semantic memory and declarative versus procedural memory.

It is fascinating to see that despite considerable experimental achievements with specific paradigms used to analyze memory function and dysfunction in healthy and ageing subjects, as well as patients with a variety of cerebral disorders affecting the hippocampus, even today important observations can only be made when straightforward clinical signs and symptoms are properly investigated and followed by specifically designed investigations. Already described in the 1960s by C. Miller Fisher and R.D. Adams, episodes of temporary amnesia are now increasingly being recognized in patients. While this syndrome was fairly similar in all of their 17 subjects, the etiology has still not been fully clarified until today [3]:

> [Patients] experienced a sudden episode of temporary amnesia, usually of a few hours duration, after which there was a complete restoration to the previous state of health. Their case reports detailed were strikingly similar and appeared to represent a distinct clinical syndrome which hereto-

fore had not been delineated in the literature. The nature of these episodes has not yet been determined but is tentatively suggested to represent a specific type of focal cerebral seizure.

With the advent of imaging in more clinical conditions, neurologists were keen to localize abnormalities in different brain areas, and the hippocampus in particular was suspected to be involved. However, studies during or immediately after the onset of transient global amnesia without loss of CA1 neurons revealed no abnormalities whatsoever. Only by chance was the first patient in our department investigated within a 48-hour delay period after the weekend, revealing punctuated lesions in the hippocampus on diffusion-weighted magnetic resonance imaging, which was then consistently observed in more than 80% of patients in subsequent studies [4]. Today this is a diagnostic confirmation of the transient and benign nature of a frightening situation (fig. 2). Surprisingly, the majority of patients suffered a serious emotional situation (funeral of a close relative or friend, excessive sports, psychogenic or organic pain and discomfort, etc.) which implicated that modulation of stress could represent a clue to affect projections to the hippocampus or vice versa.

CA1 regions of the hippocampus are particularly vulnerable to both Alzheimer's disease-type degeneration and anoxia-related dementia. In Alzheimer's disease, loss of neurons are more frequently observed than in vascular dementia, but severity of loss correlates with structure and function of subtypes. Reductions of hippocampal volume reflect loss rather than shrinkage of CA1 neurons and is eventually absent in patients with Parkinson's disease and healthy ageing. Focal anatomic and functional characteristics of the hippocampus could also play a role in the unusual distribution of lesions according to the dense neurovascular anatomy of the hippocampus.

References

1 Carlesimo GA, Piras F, Assogna F, Pontieri FE, Caltagirone C, Spalletta G: Hippocampal abnormalities and memory deficits in Parkinson disease: a multimodal imaging study. Neurology 2012;78:1939–1945.

2 Anderson P, Morris R, Amaral D, Bliss T, O'Keefe T: Historical perspective: proposed functions, biological characteristics, and neurobiological models of the hippocampus; in: The Hippocampus Book. Oxford, Oxford University Press, 2007, pp 9–36.

3 Fisher CM, Adams RD: Transient Global Amnesia. Acta Neurol Scand 1964;40(suppl 9):1–83.

4 Sedlaczek O, Hirsch JG, Grips E, Peters CN, Gass A, Wöhrle J, Hennerici M: Detection of delayed focal MR changes in the lateral hippocampus in transient global amnesia. Neurology 2004;62:2165–2170.

Prof. Dr. M.G. Hennerici
Department of Neurology, UniversitätsMedizin Mannheim
Theodor-Kutzer-Ufer 1-3
DE–68167 Mannheim (Germany)
E-Mail hennerici@neuro.ma.uni-heidelberg.de

Szabo K, Hennerici MG (eds): The Hippocampus in Clinical Neuroscience.
Front Neurol Neurosci. Basel, Karger, 2014, vol 34, pp 6–17 (DOI: 10.1159/000360925)

Anatomy of the Hippocampal Formation

Christian Schultz · Maren Engelhardt

Institute of Neuroanatomy, Center for Biomedicine and Medical Technology Mannheim (CBTM),
Medical Faculty Mannheim, Heidelberg University, Mannheim, Germany

Abstract

The hippocampus is one of several brain regions that together comprise the hippocampal formation. The hippocampal formation is a prominent C-shaped structure bulging in the floor of the temporal horn of the lateral ventricle. The hippocampus proper consists of three major subfields (CA1–CA3). The other regions that together comprise the hippocampal formation consist of the dentate gyrus, the subicular complex, and the entorhinal cortex. Based on its extrinsic connectivity, the hippocampal formation receives a vast amount of highly processed multimodal sensory information that is funneled into the hippocampal formation mainly by the entorhinal cortex. The entorhinal cortex is connected to associational neocortical areas in a reciprocal manner. Extensive hippocampal integration of sensory information is established by a largely unidirectional chain of intrinsic hippocampal projections. Our current knowledge on hippocampal connectivity and function is largely based on studies of rodents and monkeys. It still remains to be determined to which extent such neuroanatomical data of experimental animals is applicable to the human hippocampal formation.

© 2014 S. Karger AG, Basel

Gross Anatomical Features

The gross anatomical analysis of the hippocampal formation dates back to Arantius [1] who first described the appearance of human hippocampal formation and gave it the name hippocampus (derived from the Greek word for sea horse). Other authors such as Winslow [2] highlighted the resemblance of the hippocampus to a ram's horn, and Croissant de Garengeot [3] named the hippocampus Ammon's horn after an ancient Egyptian god. The term 'cornu ammonis' was introduced by the neuroanatomist Rafael Lorente de Nó [4]. In this chapter, the term 'hippocampal formation' refers to the dentate gyrus, hippocampus, subicular complex, and entorhinal cortex.

The hippocampal formation is a prominent C-shaped structure bulging in the floor of the temporal horn of the lateral ventricle (see Insausti and Amaral [5] for a comprehensive review). The human hippocampal formation has a rostrocaudal extent of approximately 5 cm. With respect to their position to the corpus callosum, the hippocampus can be divided into a precommissural, supracommissural, and retrocommissural part. Whereas the first two parts are relatively small, the retrocommissural hippocampus represents the main portion of the hippocampal formation.

The hippocampal formation is widest at its anterior extent where it bends toward the medial surface of the brain. This medial region of the hippocampal formation is known as the uncus. The number of rostrocaudal flexures in this bend of the hippocampal formation varies substantially from individual to individual and can number as many as five. The uncus shows complex images of the hippocampal formation comprised of several different hippocampal fields (detailed below). The few subtle gyri in this region are referred to as the hippocampal digitations and give this region a paw-like appearance. Accordingly, the name pes (foot) hippocampus is coined for this area. Continuing caudally, the hippocampus tapers off and bends upward around the splenium of the corpus callosum.

At the rostral limit of the lateral ventricle, the hippocampal formation (dentate gyrus, hippocampus, subicular complex) bends medially and then caudally. The dentate gyrus makes this bend most caudally, whereas the last field to make the medial bend is the subiculum. As the hippocampal formation curves dorsally to meet the retrosplenial region, the hippocampal cytoarchitecture becomes increasingly complex (see below). In principal, hippocampal fields that make up the rostral extreme of the hippocampus (i.e. the subiculum and CA1) also make up the caudal extreme. The remaining fields (dentate gyrus, CA3, and CA2) are enclosed by CA1 and the subiculum and therefore appear to end at a more rostral level than the CA1 field and subiculum. The dentate gyrus ends just caudal to the beginning of the calcarine sulcus of the occipital lobe.

Ventromedial Surface
The ventromedial surface of the temporal lobe is organized by the occipitotemporal and the collateral sulci. Rostrally, the collateral sulcus frequently coalesces with the rhinal sulcus. Together, these two sulci form the lateral border of the parahippocampal gyrus. This gyrus consists of an anterior part comprised of the entorhinal cortex and associated perirhinal cortex and the posterior parahippocampal cortex comprised of the TF and TH fields [6]. The entorhinal cortex terminates along the medial bank of the collateral sulcus. The remainder of the collateral sulcus is comprised of areas 35 and 36 of the perirhinal cortex.

A conspicuous feature of the human entorhinal cortex consists of superficial wart-like protuberances corresponding to islands of entorhinal layer II neurons. The dorsomedial aspect of the entorhinal cortex (or anterior parahippocampal gyrus) is marked by the gyrus ambiens. The rostral pole of the uncus is often designated as the gyrus uncinatus. Caudally, it is followed by the most medial bend of the dentate gyrus designated as the tail of the dentate gyrus or limbus of Giacomini. Ventrally, the uncus is limited by the rostral part of the hippocampal fissure. Caudally to the uncus, the choroidal fissure marks the medial surface of the dentate gyrus and fimbria. The hippocampal fissure separates the dentate gyrus or hippocampus from the underlying subiculum.

Caudally, the hippocampal formation merges into the retrosplenial region in the form of two obliquely oriented small gyri. The medial one is designated as the fasciola cinerea and contains the caudal part of the dentate gyrus. The lateral one – referred to as the gyrus fasciolaris – represents the terminal portion of CA3. Finally, the supracallosal tissue of the hippocampus mainly consists of remnants of the subiculum and CA1.

Dorsomedial Surface

A number of distinct cytoarchitectonic fields, including the dentate gyrus, hippocampus, and subicular cortices, are included in this region. Myelinated axons originating from pyramidal neurons of the hippocampus and subiculum travel in the white matter which sheaths the hippocampus (the alveus) and merge into the medially situated fimbria corresponding to a fringe of myelinated fibers along the medial surface of the hippocampus. The fimbria leaves the hippocampus and coalesces into the fornix which fuses with the ventral surface of the corpus callosum traveling rostrally in the lateral ventricle. The part of the fornix fused with the corpus callosum is called the crus fornicis, whereas the major rostral portion is called the body of the fornix. The descending column of the fornix is divided around the anterior commissure to form the precommissural and the postcommissural fornix. At the posterior corpus callosum (splenium), fibers of the rodent fornix form a prominent hippocampal commissure, which is often referred to as the 'psalterium' alluding to an ancient string instrument. Of note, commissural connections in the human hippocampus appear much more limited as compared to rodents [7].

Cytoarchitecture of the Hippocampal Formation

For a detailed analysis of the human hippocampal cytoarchitecture, the reader is referred to the pigmentoarchitectonic work of Braak [8] and to the comprehensive book chapter of Insausti and Amaral [5]. A variety of nomenclatures have been used to label the portions of the hippocampal formation, depending on what species is considered. Based on the nomenclature of Lorente de Nó [4], the hippocampus is divided into four fields designated as CA1–CA4. However, as suggested by Insausti and Amaral [5] the term CA4 should be omitted since these neurons should probably belong to the hilar region of CA3 (fig. 1a; detailed below).

Dentate Gyrus

The dentate gyrus forms the medial-most part of the cerebral cortex. At the cytoarchitectural level the dentate gyrus is a trilaminate cortical region (fig. 1a). At mid-rostrocaudal levels of the hippocampal formation, the dentate gyrus forms a typical

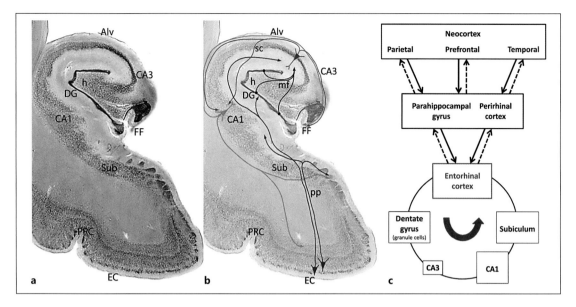

Fig. 1. a Low-power view of the human hippocampal formation. For purpose of cytoarchitectonic investigation, the 100-μm thick section was stained for lipofuscin pigment (aldehyde fuchsin) and for Nissl material (Darrow red). **b** Intrinsic hippocampal connectivity superimposed upon a section of the human hippocampal formation. See text for further description. **c** Pattern of cortical and intrinsic connectivity of the hippocampal formation. Note the reciprocal flow of cortical information converging via the parahippocampal gyrus and perirhinal cortex upon the entorhinal cortex. By comparison, the intrinsic hippocampal circuitry is arranged in a largely undirectional manner (see text). Alv = Alveus; CA1–CA3 = sectors of the Ammons horn; DG = dentate gyrus; EC = entorhinal cortex; FF = fimbria/fornix; h = hilus of the dentate gyrus; mf = mossy fibers; pp = perforant pathway; sub = subiculum; PRC = perirhinal cortex; sc = Schaffer collaterals.

C-shaped structure that is separated ventrally from CA1 and the subiculum by the hippocampal fissure. The principal cell layer of the dentate gyrus is densely packed with somata of granule cells (approx. 15×10^6 neurons) [9]. The spiny dendrites of these cells branch extensively in the dentate molecular layer. Human dentate granule cells also extend basal dendrites into the subjacent polymorphic layer [10]. The granule cell and molecular layers together represent the fascia dentata.

The third and innermost layer of the dentate gyrus is called the polymorphic layer or hilus and sometimes referred to as the hippocampal field CA4. However, the hilus cells project only to the dentate gyrus [11]. Therefore, the polymorphic layer most often is considered as a part of the dentate gyrus. Close to the hilus, a fraction of the pyramidal cell layer is enclosed by the granule cell layer. There is no obvious cytoarchitectonic or connectional difference between these neurons and adjacent CA3 pyramidal neurons [5]. Therefore, the term CA4 for these neurons should be avoided. Instead, all pyramidal neurons close to the dentate hilus should be considered as constituents of CA3.

Hippocampus

The human hippocampus can be divided into the fields CA3, CA2, and CA1 [4, 5]. These hippocampal fields have essentially one cellular layer, the pyramidal cell layer. The limiting surface with the ventricular lumen is formed by axons of the pyramidal cells and is called the alveus. Between it and the pyramidal cell layer, the stratum oriens mainly contains the basal dendrites of the pyramidal cells as well as several types of interneurons. The region superficial to the pyramidal cell layer (toward the hippocampal fissure) contains the apical dendrites of the pyramidal cells and a number of interneurons. This region has historically been divided into (1) the stratum lucidum, (2) the stratum radiatum, and (3) the stratum lacunosum-moleculare corresponding to the most superficial portion (adjacent to the hippocampal fissure) of this region.

In principal, the apical dendrites of pyramidal neurons make up the stratum radiatum, whereas the stratum lacunosum-moleculare contains the terminal branches of these dendrites. At the opposite pole, basal dendrites of pyramidal neurons ramify in the stratum oriens. Axons of pyramidal neurons enter the outermost subependymal fiber layer (alveus).

In the stratum lucidum of CA3, the mossy fibers travel and form synapses with proximal dendrites just above the pyramidal cell layer of CA3. In the human hippocampus a fraction of the mossy fibers also travel within the CA3 pyramidal cell layer. Stratum lucidum is absent in CA2 and CA1, which do not receive mossy fiber input.

The hallmark of CA3 neurons is that their proximal dendrites are contacted by mossy fibers which correspond to the dentate granule cell axons. The mossy fibers traverse the stratum lucidum immediately above the CA3 pyramidal cell layer. In the stratum radiatum, apical dendrites of CA3 and CA2 neurons receive associational projections from other rostrocaudal levels as well as cholinergic and histaminergic input from septal nuclei and supramammillary regions, respectively. In CA1, the projections from CA3 and CA2 – the so-called Schaffer collaterals – terminate in the stratum radiatum and stratum oriens. The perforant pathway projection from the entorhinal cortex to the dentate gyrus travels, in part, in the stratum lacunosum-moleculare of the hippocampus and makes en passant synapses on the distal apical dendrites of the hippocampal pyramidal cells. As compared to the neighboring fields (in particular CA1), CA3 is relatively insensitive to pathology corresponding to the so-called resistant sector of classical neuropathology [12].

The CA2 region has a relatively compact and narrow pyramidal cell layer. In routine preparations of the human hippocampus, the borders of CA2 are difficult to establish. The primate CA2 region has a distinct connectivity with prominent histaminergic input from the hypothalamic tuberomammillary nucleus [13].

Phylogenetically, CA1 is a progressive subfield of the hippocampus [14]. In particular, the pyramidal cell laxer of CA1 becomes thicker and more heterogeneous in monkeys and humans as compared to rodents. Stereological studies estimate the total number of CA1 neurons as approximately 14×10^6 [9]. The appearance of CA1 varies along its transverse and rostrocaudal axes. Based on pigmentoarchitectonic studies, the human CA1 pyramidal cell layer can be subdivided into an outer and inner pyramidal cell layer [15]. Close to the CA2 border, the CA1 pyramidal cell layer is at its thinnest, and the cells of both sublayers appear most tightly packed. The border of CA1 with CA2 is ill-defined because some CA2 pyramidal cells appear to extend over the emerging CA1 pyramidal cell layer. The pyramidal cell layer of CA1 overlaps that of the subiculum in an oblique manner.

Subiculum

As described, the subiculum and CA1 overlap at their border, forming a complex transitional zone. In principal, the subiculum can be divided into three layers. Superficially, there is a wide molecular layer into which the apical dendrites of the subicular pyramidal cells extend. The pyramidal cell layer of the subiculum can be further divided into an external and internal sublayer [16]. The cells of the external cell layer contain a conspicuous accumulation of lipofuscin pigment in their apical dendrites. The subiculum gives rise to major subcortical projections to the septal complex, nucleus accumbens, anterior thalamus, and mammillary nuclei, as well as projections to the entorhinal cortex (detailed below). The presubiculum consists of a single, superficially located cellular layer (layer II), containing densely packed modified pyramidal neurons. The parasubiculum also contains a single cellular layer that is difficult to differentiate from the presubiculum.

Entorhinal Cortex

The term 'entorhinal cortex' is synonymous for Brodmann area 28. The entorhinal cortex extends rostrally to about the midlevel of the amygdala and caudally to the level of the anterior limit of the lateral geniculate nucleus (fig. 1a). Phylogenetically, the primate entorhinal cortex has undergone substantial differentiation [14]. Up to seven cytoarchitectonic fields can be distinguished in monkeys. In humans up to eight fields can be separated [17]. Laterally, the deep layers of the entorhinal cortex extend further than the superficial layers. Thereby, a distinct oblique border between the entorhinal cortex and adjacent area 35 is generated. This oblique transition zone has also been designated as the 'transentorhinal zone' [8]. Interestingly, transentorhinal neurons are highly susceptible to the earliest preclinical stages of Alzheimer-related neurofibrillary pathology [18]. Caudally, the primate entorhinal cortex is continuous with the parahippocampal gyrus (fields TH and TF).

The laminar organization of the entorhinal cortex is distinct from other neocortical regions. In principal, six entorhinal layers can be distinguished (fig. 1a). Layer I is an acellular or plexiform layer. Layer II is highly characteristic of the entorhinal cortex. It is made up of islands of modified pyramidal and stellate cells [8]. The cell islands of layer II form small protrusions on the entorhinal surface that can be observed with the unaided eye. These wart-like protrusions ('verrucae hippocampi') provide a useful macroscopic indication of the entorhinal location. Layer III contains a homogeneous population of pyramidal cells. Dendrites of layer III pyramidal neurons pass through the space between layer II cell islands [19]. Beneath layer III, a distinctive cell-sparse lamina – the so-called lamina dissecans – is found. This lamina highlights the virtual absence of a layer IV (internal granule cell layer). Accordingly, the cells subjacent to the lamina dissecans are designated as layer V. Layer VI of the entorhinal cortex is not easily distinguished from layer V.

Hippocampal Connectivity

Intrinsic Hippocampal Circuit
In principal, the intrinsic flow of hippocampal information follows a serial and largely unidirectional and glutamatergic (excitatory) path that ultimately forms part of a closed circuit (fig. 1b, c). In this intrinsic chain of connections, the dentate gyrus represents the first major gateway. The dentate gyrus itself receives major input from layer II cells of the entorhinal cortex via the so-called perforant path [20]. The perforant path travels caudally from the entorhinal cortex (via the angular bundle) and perforates the subiculum and hippocampus. Specifically, entorhinal layer II neurons project to the outer two thirds of the molecular layer of the dentate gyrus and stratum lacunosum-moleculare of CA3, whereas entorhinal layer III neurons project to CA1 and the subiculum.

The dentate granule cells project via their distinctive axons, the mossy fibers, upon cells of the subjacent dentate polymorphic layer and – more importantly – onto proximal dendrites of CA3 pyramidal neurons. The precise connectivity of the heterogeneous neurons of the polymorphic layer is largely unknown. However, these neurons give rise to both local and associational projections [21]. In marked contrast to rodents, only sparse commissural projections originate from primate dentate polymorphic neurons [7, 22]. One class of cell, the mossy cell, gives rise to a glutamatergic associational system of fibers that terminates in the inner one third of the dentate molecular layer [23]. This projection may help to connect different rostrocaudal levels of the dentate gyrus. With regard to the vast literature on hippocampal interneurons, the reader is referred to the review of Freund and Buzsáki [21].

Collaterals of single CA3 pyramidal cells project to other levels of CA3, as well as to CA1 and to subcortical regions (septal nuclei; detailed below). Importantly, CA3 cells also give rise to the major input system to CA1 via the Schaffer collaterals, which terminate throughout the stratum radiatum and stratum oriens of CA1 [24, 25]. In nonhuman primates this important projection extends for more than two thirds along the longitudinal axis of the hippocampus [26]. To a lesser extent CA3 also gives rise to associational fibers targeting other rostrocaudal levels of CA3.

In contrast to CA3, CA1 pyramidal cells do not project significantly to other CA1 levels. Instead, CA1 pyramidal cells project predominantly to the subiculum. The subiculum, in turn, projects to the pre- and parasubiculum and all three components of the subicular cortices finally project to the entorhinal cortex [25, 27, 28].

Extrinsic Connections

Extrinsic input which modulates the hippocampal circuitry arises from (1) various cortical areas, (2) the amygdaloid complex, (3) the medial septal region, (4) the thalamus, (5) the supramamillary region, and (6) monoaminergic brainstem nuclei. The classical view of the extrinsic connectivity of the hippocampal formation is based on studies of Papez [29]. This view suggests that the hippocampus receives sensory information from a variety of cortical regions and serves to forward this information through the fimbria and fornix to the mammillary nuclei where appropriate emotional responses are finally evoked. It is now clear, however, that the subiculum provides the vast majority of fibers travelling via the fornix to the mammillary complex. Moreover, the fornix is not the sole output pathway of the primate hippocampal system. In this context, the subiculum is a major source for neocortical output of the hippocampal formation, directed to polymodal association cortices [30–34]. Likewise, the entorhinal cortex projects to neighboring cortices such as the perirhinal and parahippocampal cortices and to more distant regions such as the orbitofrontal cortex. The hippocampal formation can also influence a variety of brain regions through nonfimbrial projections to the amygdaloid complex and striatum.

Cortical Connections

Corticohippocampal projections mainly serve to convey multimodal sensory information into the hippocampal formation (fig. 1c). In the medial temporal lobe, this sensory information is further processed along a hierarchical chain represented by (1) the perirhinal and posterior parahippocampal cortices, (2) the entorhinal cortex, and (3) the hippocampal formation itself. Specifically, the TF and TH areas of the posterior parahippocampal gyrus, the perirhinal cortex (area 35), and the temporal polar cortex project to the lateral entorhinal cortex [35–37]. Cortical areas projecting directly to the entorhinal cortex include the superior temporal gyrus, the ventral (agranular) insular cortex, the posterior orbitofrontal cortex (area 13), the dorsolateral frontal cortex (areas 9, 10, and 46), the medial frontal cortex (areas 25 and 32), the cingulate cortex (areas 24 and 23), and the caudally adjacent retrosplenial cortex (areas 29 and 30). Insausti et al. [37] estimated that two thirds of all the cortical input of the entorhinal cortex originate in the surrounding multimodal sensory association cortices. Only limited hippocampal input appears to originate directly from unimodal sensory cortices [37–39]. However, the entorhinal cortex does receive some olfactory information originating from the olfactory bulb or from the prepirifom cortex [40].

The vast majority of cortical areas that project to the entorhinal cortex receive reciprocal projections. Thus, entorhinal projections are directed towards the adjacent perirhinal cortex, the temporal polar cortex, the caudal parahippocampal gyrus, and the caudal cingulate gyrus [41, 42]. Based on such connectivity, the hippocampal formation exerts control over widespread regions of the temporal, parietal, and frontal lobes. It has been emphasized that the parahippocampal gyrus, in particular, projects to virtually all the associational cortices of the primate brain [6]. With regard to non-entorhinal cortical efferents, retrograde tracing techniques in the primate brain have shown that CA1 and the subicular complex give rise to nonentorhinal neocortical output directed to polymodal association cortices [32–34]. It should be noted that the subiculum also receives direct neocortical input. Thus, the temporal polar cortex, the perirhinal cortex, and the parahippocampal gyrus project to one or more divisions of the subicular complex [43]. In addition to its subcortical projections to the anterior thalamus and mammillary nuclei, Rosene and Van Hoesen [25] demonstrated that the monkey subicular cortices project to several cortical fields, including the perirhinal cortex, the parahippocampal gyrus, the caudal cingulate gyrus, and the medial frontal and medial orbitofrontal cortices. The nonhuman primate subicular cortices were shown to reciprocate the projections to most of these areas [25, 32, 33].

Subcortical Connections

The fimbria and fornix form the classical efferent system of the hippocampal formation. The human fornix contains about 1.2 million fibers [44]. The precommissural fornix primarily innervates the lateral septal nucleus, and arises mainly from the hippocampus proper and to a lesser extent from the subiculum and entorhinal cortex [45, 46]. The cells of CA3, which project to the septal complex, also give rise to the Schaffer collaterals to CA1. The nucleus accumbens is also contacted by fibers of the fornix that arise in the subiculum and entorhinal cortex [47, 48].

Of note, the subicular complex – rather than the cornu ammonis – is the major source of the postcommissural fiber system of the fornix [49]. Accordingly, fibers originating in the subiculum/presubiculum provide the major extrinsic input to the mammillary nuclei [25, 48, 50].

Major connections also exist between the hippocampal formation and the amygdala [40]. The lateral nucleus of the amygdala projects to layer III of the lateral entorhinal cortex. In primates, the lateral and basal nuclei also project to the entorhinal cortex and there are additional projections from the accessory basal nucleus to the subiculum. The subiculum reciprocally projects to the basal nucleus, while the entorhinal cortex projects to both the basal and lateral nuclei.

Other prominent subcortical structures that project to the hippocampal formation include the medial septal complex. In rodents, the partially cholinergic medial septal projection arises from the medial septal nucleus and the diagonal band of Broca [51]. Septal fibers are most prominent in the dentate gyrus and CA3. Approximately 50% of the cells in the medial septal nucleus that project to the hippocampal formation are cholinergic [52]. Noncholinergic septal neurons that project to the hippocampus presumably are GABAergic [53]. The hippocampal formation receives major hypothalamic input from the supramammillary area [54–56]. This supramammillary projection terminates via the fornix in all hippocampal fields, but is most prominent in the dentate gyrus, in fields CA2 and CA3 of the hippocampus, and in the rostral entorhinal cortex.

Reciprocal connections between the hippocampal formation and the hypothalamus are established by the subiculum projecting to the medial and lateral mammillary nuclei. In addition, there are perifornical cells that project to the hippocampal formation.

The hippocampal formation also receives substantial projections from thalamic nuclei which primarily arise from the anterior thalamic complex and lateral dorsal nucleus [50, 54, 56], forming a part of the so-called circuit of Papez. The midline thalamic nuclei (paraventricular nucleus, nucleus centralis medialis, nucleus reuniens) also project to the hippocampal formation [56].

With regard to brainstem innervation, a major noradrenergic input arises from the locus coeruleus [55]. The mesencephalic raphe nuclei give rise to a major serotonergic innervation [57]. In addition, all components of the hippocampal formation receive dopaminergic projections from the ventral tegmental area [56, 58].

Commissural Connections

Prominent hippocampal commissures primarily exist in rodents [58]. In monkeys, only the uncus and the associated dentate gyrus are interconnected by commissural fibers. This contrasts markedly with the rodent brain, where both CA3 and CA1 of the entire hippocampus receive a strong, topographically organized projection from the opposite CA3, and the dentate gyrus receives a major input from cells of the contralateral polymorphic layer [7]. As in the rat, the monkey presubiculum gives rise to a substantial commissural projection that terminates in layer III of the contralateral entorhinal cortex. In primates this projection may constitute the major link between the hippocampal formations of the two sides. Gloor et al. [22] studied human postmortem brains and identified a dorsal hippocampal commissure that had an appearance similar to that of the monkey.

This brief overview shall suffice as a neuroanatomical introduction for the subsequent chapters. The reader of this book should be aware that our current knowledge on hippocampal neuroanatomy and function is largely based on studies of rodents and monkeys. It will be a major challenge for future research to precisely determine to which extent such data also applies to the human hippocampal formation.

References

1 Arantius G: De humano foetu. Ejusdem anatomicorum observationum liber, etc. Venice, 1587, pp 44–45.
2 Winslow JB: Exposition anatomique de la structure du corps humain. Paris, Desprez et Desessartz, 1732.
3 Croissant de Garengeot RJ: Splanchnologie ou l'anatomie de visceres, ed 2. Paris, Osmont, 1742.
4 Lorente de Nó R: Studies on the structure of the cerebral cortex. II. Continuation of the study of the ammonic system. J Psychol Neurol 1934, pp 113–177.
5 Insausti AM, Amaral DG: Hippocampal formation; in Mai JK, Paxinos G (eds): The Human Nervous System, ed 3. San Diego, Academic Press, 2012, pp 896–942.

6 Van Hoesen G, Garry W: The parahippocampal gyrus: new observations regarding its cortical connections in the monkey. Trends Neurosci 1982;5:345–350.

7 Amaral DG, Insausti R, Cowan WM: The commissural connections of the monkey hippocampal formation. J Comp Neurol 1984;224:307–336.

8 Braak H: Architectonics of the human telencephalic cortex. Berlin, Springer, 1980.

9 West MJ, Coleman PD, Flood DG, Troncoso JC: Differences in the pattern of hippocampal neuronal loss in normal ageing and Alzheimer's disease. Lancet 1994;344:769–772.

10 Seress L, Mrzljak L: Basal dendrites of granule cells are normal features of the fetal and adult dentate gyrus of both monkey and human hippocampal formations. Brain Res 1987;405:169–174.

11 Laurberg S, Sorensen KE: Associational and commissural collaterals of neurons in the hippocampal formation (hilus fasciae dentatae and subfield CA3). Brain Res 1981;212:287–300.

12 Sloviter RS: The functional organization of the hippocampal dentate gyrus and its relevance to the pathogenesis of temporal lobe epilepsy. Ann Neurol 1994;35:640–654.

13 Veazey C, Amaral DG, Cowan WM: The morphology and connections of the posterior hypothalamus in the cynomolgous monkey. II. Efferent connections. J Comp Neurol 1982;207:135–156.

14 Stephan H: Evolutionary trends in limbic structures. Neurosci Biobehav Rev 1983;7:367–374.

15 Braak H: On the structure of the human archicortex. I. The cornu ammonis. A golgi and pigmentarchitectonic study. Cell Tissue Res 1974;152:349–383.

16 Braak H: Pigmentarchitecture of the human cortex cerebri. II. Subiculum (in German). Z Zellforsch Mikrosk Anat 1972;131:235–254.

17 Insausti R, Tunon T, Sobreviela T, Insausti AM, Gonzalo LM: The human entorhinal cortex: a cytoarchitectonic analysis. J Comp Neurol 1995;355:171–198.

18 Braak E, Braak H, Mandelkow EM: A sequence of cytoskeleton changes related to the formation of neurofibrillary tangles and neuropil threads. Acta Neuropathol 1994;87:554–567.

19 Carboni AA, Lavelle WG, Barnes CL, Cipolloni PB: Neurons of the lateral entorhinal cortex of the rhesus monkey: a golgi, histochemical, and immunocytochemical characterization. J Comp Neurol 1990;291:583–608.

20 Witter MP, Amaral DG: Entorhinal cortex of the monkey: V. Projections to the dentate gyrus, hippocampus, and subicular complex. J Comp Neurol 1991;307:437–459.

21 Freund TF, Buzsáki G: Interneurons of the hippocampus. Hippocampus 1996;6:347–470.

22 Gloor P, Salanova V, Olivier A, Quesney LF: The human dorsal hippocampal commissure. An anatomically identifiable and functional pathway. Brain 1993;116:1249–1273.

23 Soriano E, Frotscher M: Mossy cells of the rat fascia dentata are glutamate-immunoreactive. Hippocampus 1994;4:65–69.

24 Ishizuka N, Weber J, Amaral DG: Organization of intrahippocampal projections originating from CA3 pyramidal cells in the rat. J Comp Neurol 1990;295:580–623.

25 Rosene DL, Van Hoesen GW: Hippocampal efferents reach widespread areas of cerebral cortex and amygdala in the rhesus monkey. Science 1977;198:315–317.

26 Kondo H, Lavenex P, Amaral DG: Intrinsic connections of the macaque monkey hippocampal formation: II. CA3 connections. J Comp Neurol 2009;515:349–377.

27 Beckstead RM: Afferent connections of the entorhinal area in the rat as demonstrated by retrograde cell-labeling with horseradish peroxidase. Brain Res 1978;152:249–264.

28 Finch DM, Nowlin NL, Babb TL: Demonstration of axonal projections of neurons in the rat hippocampus and subiculum by intracellular injection of HRP. Brain Res 1983;271:201–216.

29 Papez JW: A proposed mechanism of emotion. Arch Neurol Psychiatry 1937;38:725–743.

30 Barbas H, Blatt GJ: Topographically specific hippocampal projections target functionally distinct prefrontal areas in the rhesus monkey. Hippocampus 1995;5:511–533.

31 Blatt GJ, Rosene DL: Organization of direct hippocampal efferent projections to the cerebral cortex of the rhesus monkey: projections from CA1, prosubiculum, and subiculum to the temporal lobe. J Comp Neurol 1998;392:92–114.

32 Ding SL, Van Hoesen G, Rockland KS: Inferior parietal lobule projections to the presubiculum and neighboring ventromedial temporal cortical areas. J Comp Neurol 2000;425:510–530.

33 Yukie M: Connections between the medial temporal cortex and the CA1 subfield of the hippocampal formation in the Japanese monkey (*Macaca fuscata*). J Comp Neurol 2000;423:282–298.

34 Insausti R, Munoz M: Cortical projections of the non-entorhinal hippocampal formation in the cynomolgus monkey (*Macaca fascicularis*). Eur J Neurosci 2001;14:435–451.

35 Van Hoesen G, Pandya DN: Some connections of the entorhinal (area 28) and perirhinal (area 35) cortices of the rhesus monkey. I. Temporal lobe afferents. Brain Res 1975;95:1–24.

36 Van Hoesen G, Pandya DN, Butters N: Some connections of the entorhinal (area 28) and perirhinal (area 35) cortices of the rhesus monkey. II. Frontal lobe afferents. Brain Res 1975;95:25–38.

37 Insausti R, Amaral DG, Cowan WM: The entorhinal cortex of the monkey: II. Cortical afferents. J Comp Neurol 1987;264:356–395.

38 Mohedano-Moriano A, Pro-Sistiaga P, Arroyo-Jimenez MM, Artacho-Perula E, Insausti AM, Marcos P, Cebada-Sanchez S, Martinez-Ruiz J, Munoz M, Blaizot X, Martinez-Marcos A, Amaral DG, Insausti R: Topographical and laminar distribution of cortical input to the monkey entorhinal cortex. J Anat 2007;211:250–260.

39 Mohedano-Moriano A, Martinez-Marcos A, Pro-Sistiaga P, Blaizot X, Arroyo-Jimenez MM, Marcos P, Artacho-Perula E, Insausti R: Convergence of unimodal and polymodal sensory input to the entorhinal cortex in the fascicularis monkey. Neuroscience 2008;151:255–271.

40 Krettek JE, Price JL: Projections from the amygdaloid complex and adjacent olfactory structures to the entorhinal cortex and to the subiculum in the rat and cat. J Comp Neurol 1977;172:723–752.

41 Van Hoesen GW: Anatomy of the medial temporal lobe. Magn Reson Imaging 1995;13:1047–1055.

42 Suzuki WA, Amaral DG: Topographic organization of the reciprocal connections between the monkey entorhinal cortex and the perirhinal and parahippocampal cortices. J Neurosci 1994;14:1856–1877.

43 Van Hoesen GW, Rosene DL, Mesulam MM: Subicular input from temporal cortex in the rhesus monkey. Science 1979;205:608–610.

44 Powell TP, Guillery RW, Cowan WM: A quantitative study of the fornixmamillo-thalamic system. J Anat 1957;91:419–437.

45 Alonso A, Kohler C: A study of the reciprocal connections between the septum and the entorhinal area using anterograde and retrograde axonal transport methods in the rat brain. J Comp Neurol 1984;225:327–343.

46 Siegel A, Ohgami S, Edinger H: Projections of the hippocampus to the septal area in the squirrel monkey. Brain Res 1975;99:247–260.

47 Groenewegen HJ, Room P, Witter MP, Lohman AH: Cortical afferents of the nucleus accumbens in the cat, studied with anterograde and retrograde transport techniques. Neuroscience 1982;7:977–996.

48 Swanson LW, Cowan WM: An autoradiographic study of the organization of the efferent connections of the hippocampal formation in the rat. J Comp Neurol 1977;172:49–84.

49 Swanson LW, Cowan WM: Hippocampo-hypothalamic connections: origin in subicular cortex, not Ammon's horn. Science 1975;189:303–304.

50 Irle E, Markowitsch HJ: Single and combined lesions of the cats thalamic mediodorsal nucleus and the mamillary bodies lead to severe deficits in the acquisition of an alternation task. Behav Brain Res 1982;6:147–165.

51 Milner TA, Amaral DG: Evidence for a ventral septal projection to the hippocampal formation of the rat. Exp Brain Res 1984;55:579–585.

52 Mesulam MM, Mufson EJ, Levey AI, Wainer BH: Cholinergic innervation of cortex by the basal forebrain: cytochemistry and cortical connections of the septal area, diagonal band nuclei, nucleus basalis (substantia innominata), and hypothalamus in the rhesus monkey. J Comp Neurol 1983;214:170–197.

53 Köhler C, Chan-Palay V, Wu JY: Septal neurons containing glutamic acid decarboxylase immunoreactivity project to the hippocampal region in the rat brain. Anat Embryol (Berl) 1984;169:41–44.

54 Amaral DG, Cowan WM: Subcortical afferents to the hippocampal formation in the monkey. J Comp Neurol 1980;189:573–591.

55 Segal M, Landis S: Afferents to the hippocampus of the rat studied with the method of retrograde transport of horseradish peroxidase. Brain Res 1974;78:1–15.

56 Insausti R, Amaral DG, Cowan WM: The entorhinal cortex of the monkey: III. Subcortical afferents. J Comp Neurol 1987;264:396–408.

57 Köhler C, Steinbusch H: Identification of serotonin and non-serotonin-containing neurons of the midbrain raphe projecting to the entorhinal area and the hippocampal formation. A combined immunohistochemical and fluorescent retrograde tracing study in the rat brain. Neuroscience 1982;7:951–975.

58 Swanson LW, Sawchenko PE, Cowan WM: Evidence that the commissural, associational and septal projections of the regio inferior of the hippocampus arise from the same neurons. Brain Res 1980;197:207–212.

Prof. Dr. med. Christian Schultz
Institute of Neuroanatomy, Center for Biomedicine and Medical Technology Mannheim (CBTM)
Medical Faculty Mannheim/Heidelberg University
Ludolf-Krehl Strasse 13-17, DE–68167 Mannheim (Germany)
E-Mail christian.schultz@medma.uni-heidelberg.de

Szabo K, Hennerici MG (eds): The Hippocampus in Clinical Neuroscience.
Front Neurol Neurosci. Basel, Karger, 2014, vol 34, pp 18–25 (DOI: 10.1159/000356440)

Structure and Vascularization of the Human Hippocampus

Laurent Tatu[a, b] · Fabrice Vuillier[b, c]

Departments of [a]Neuromuscular Diseases, [b]Anatomy, and [c]Neurology, CHU Besançon, University of Franche-Comté, Besançon, France

Abstract

The hippocampus is a temporal brain structure belonging to the limbic lobe and is fundamentally involved in memory processing, learning, and emotions. It consists of two allocortex laminae: the gyrus dentatus and the cornu ammonis, one rolled up inside the other, creating a bulge in the temporal horn of the lateral ventricle. Arterial vascularization of the hippocampus is dependent on the collateral branches of the posterior cerebral artery and the anterior choroidal artery, forming the network of superficial hippocampal arteries that in turn lead to deep intrahippocampal arteries. Venous vascularization is provided by the intrahippocampal veins, which drain into the superficial hippocampal veins. Knowledge of anatomical organization and vascularization of the hippocampus is essential to understanding its dysfunctions and its appearance on MRI.

© 2014 S. Karger AG, Basel

The hippocampus is a temporal brain structure belonging to the limbic lobe. Terminological discussions have complicated its anatomical definition, but it is now accepted that the hippocampus consists of two allocortex laminae: the gyrus dentatus and the cornu ammonis, one rolled up inside the other, creating a bulge in the temporal horn of the lateral ventricle [1]. The hippocampus is fundamentally involved in memory processing, learning, and emotions. Knowledge of its anatomical organization and its vascularization is essential to understanding its dysfunctions and its appearance on MRI. This chapter presents a global approach to the morphology of this structure and the main principles of its vascularization.

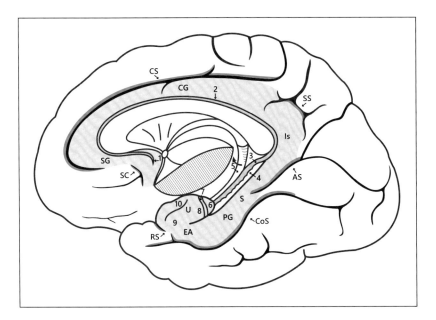

Fig. 1. Inferomedial view of the right hemisphere. The limbic lobe (gray) is delimited by the limbic fissure, which is formed by the subcallosal sulcus (SC), the cingulate sulcus (CS), the subparietal sulcus (SS), the anterior calcarine sulcus (AS), the collateral sulcus (CoS), and the rhinal sulcus (RS). The limbic gyrus comprises the subcallosal gyrus (SG), the cingulate gyrus (CG), the isthmus (Is), and the parahippocampal gyrus, which in turn includes the uncus (U), the entorhinal area (EA), and a narrow part, the subiculum (S). 1 = Prehippocampal rudiment; 2 = indusium griseum; 3 = cornu ammonis; 4 = gyrus dentatus; 5 = fimbria; 6 = uncal apex; 7 = band of Giacomini; 8 = uncinatus gyrus; 9 = ambient gyrus; 10 = semilunar gyrus.

Location of the Hippocampus

The hippocampus is a major part of the limbic lobe. The lobe is on the medial aspect of the cerebral hemisphere, separated from the rest of the cortex by the limbic fissure. It is divided into two gyri: the limbic gyrus and the intralimbic gyrus. It belongs to the intralimbic gyrus, which in turn comprises three segments named according to their position relative to the corpus callosum. The anterior segment, located in the septal region, is called the prehippocampal rudiment. Continuing from this is the superior segment, the indusium griseum, which is located on the superior surface of the corpus callosum. The inferior segment, the largest part of the intralimbic gyrus, is the hippocampus (fig. 1) [1, 2]. The hippocampus is often associated with the amygdala, a complex nucleus with which it is in direct contact and which is involved in olfaction and limbic functions. However, the amygdala is not part of the hippocampus.

The hippocampus is arc shaped and sagittally oriented, with a dilated anterior segment and a narrow posterior segment. In adults, the hippocampus is 4–5 cm long and

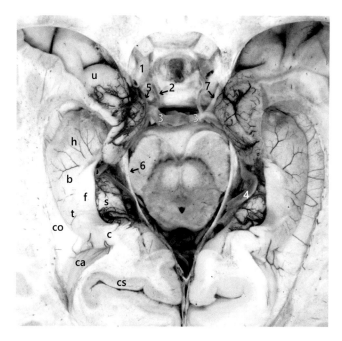

Fig. 2. Superior view of the hippocampus (horizontal section of the upper mesencephalon; the temporal horns of the lateral ventricles have been opened and the choroid plexuses removed). h = Hippocampal head; b = hippocampal body; t = hippocampal tail; f = fimbria; c = crus of fornix; s = subiculum; u = uncus; co = collateral eminence; ca = calcar avis; cs = calcarine sulcus; 1 = internal carotid artery; 2 = posterior communicating artery; 3 = posterior cerebral artery (P1 segment); 4 = posterior cerebral artery (P2 segment); 5 = anterior choroidal artery; 6 = free edge of the tentorium cerebelli; 7 = oculomotor nerve.

around 1 cm wide. It comprises three parts, the head, body, and tail, which each have a ventricular part located in the temporal horn of the lateral ventricle and an extra-ventricular part on the medial surface of the temporal lobe on the parahippocampal gyrus and uncus (fig. 2).

Hippocampal Configuration

The hippocampus is a structure made of two interlocking allocortex laminae, the dentate gyrus and the cornu ammonis. The intraventricular aspect of the hippocampus is covered by a thin layer of white matter called the alveus, which contains afferent and efferent hippocampal fibers and forms the floor of the temporal horn of the lateral ventricle (fig. 3).

The cornu ammonis is usually divided into four cortical fields: CA1, CA2, CA3, and CA4. This division is based on the cellular morphology of the cortical neurons. CA1 continues from the cortex of the parahippocampal gyrus at the subiculum, which

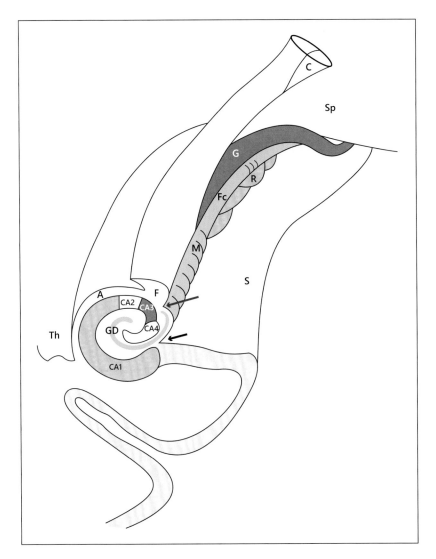

Fig. 3. Configuration of the hippocampal body and tail. GD = Gyrus dentatus; S = subiculum; Sp = splenium of the corpus callosum; Th = temporal horn of the lateral ventricle; A = alveus; F = fimbria; M = margo denticulatus; C = crus of fornix; Fc = fasciola cinerea; G = gyrus fasciolaris; R = gyrus of Andreas Retzius. The black arrow indicates the hippocampal sulcus, and the red arrow indicates the fimbriodentate sulcus.

is separated from the hippocampus by the hippocampal sulcus. The fields of the cornu ammonis have also been classified according to their susceptibility to hypoxia: CA1 is considered to be a sector vulnerable to hypoxia while CA3 is considered to be more resistant. The relative size of these four cortical fields varies depending on the hippocampal segments. The gyrus dentatus, the second allocortex lamina, owes its name to its toothed appearance. It is U-shaped and fits into the CA4 segment of the cornu ammonis. The fimbria, the principal hippocampal efferent pathway, gradually separates from the hippocampus as the crus of fornix. The gyrus dentatus and fimbria are separated by the fimbriodentate sulcus.

According to Duvernoy [1], it is possible to describe the extra- and intraventricular parts of the hippocampus. The hippocampal head is the dilated anterior segment of the hippocampus. Its ventricular part consists of 3–4 sagittal digitationes. Like the rest of the hippocampus, subependymal veins cover its surface. The extraventricular part of the hippocampal head corresponds to the posterior part of the uncus. It is formed by the uncal apex (which belongs to the cornu ammonis), the band of Giacomini (which is a segment of the gyrus dentatus), and the gyrus uncinatus (which continues to the gyrus ambiens, an anterior part of the uncus; fig. 1).

The hippocampal body is an element of the floor of the temporal horn of the lateral ventricle. Also covered by subependymal veins, it is bordered medially by the fimbria and laterally by the collateral eminence marking the ventricular protrusion of the collateral sulcus. The extraventricular part of the hippocampal body is separated from the subiculum by the hippocampal sulcus. It includes the margo denticulatus, the superficial and crenelated part of the gyrus dentatus. The margo denticulatus is covered in part by the fimbria, which ascends to join the crus of fornix. It is separated from the fimbria by the fimbriodentate sulcus (fig. 3).

The hippocampal tail is the narrow posterior part of the hippocampal arc. Its ventricular part forms the floor of the ventricular atrium. It is in medial contact with the fimbria. The extraventricular part of the hippocampal tail comprises the margo denticulatus, which gradually narrows to form the fasciola cinerea. The fimbria progressively separates from the hippocampal tail to reveal the gyrus fasciolaris, composed of CA3. CA1 also appears at the tail in the form of rounded bulges called the gyri of Andreas Retzius (fig. 3).

Arterial Vascularization of the Hippocampus

Arterial vascularization of the hippocampus is dependent on the collateral branches of the posterior cerebral artery and the anterior choroidal artery. These collateral branches form the network of superficial hippocampal arteries that in turn lead to deep intrahippocampal arteries located intraparenchymally.

Superficial Hippocampal Arteries

In its perimesencephalic segment, opposite to the crural and ambient cisterns (P2 segment), the posterior cerebral artery leads to the inferior temporal arteries (anterior, medial, and posterior), the posterolateral choroidal arteries, and the splenial arteries [3]. From these collateral arteries arise the superficial hippocampal arteries [4, 5]. In

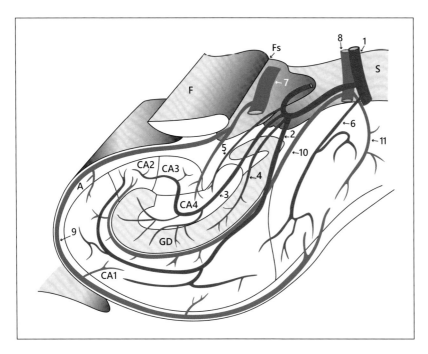

Fig. 4. Intrahippocampal vascularization. A = Alveus; F = fimbria; Fs = fimbriodentate sulcus; S = subiculum; GD = gyrus dentatus; 1 = superficial hippocampal artery; 2 = large ventral hippocampal artery; 3 = large dorsal hippocampal artery; 4 = small ventral hippocampal artery; 5 = small dorsal hippocampal artery; 6 = subiculum arteries; 7 = venous arch of the fimbriodentate sulcus; 8 = venous arch of the hippocampal sulcus; 9 = subependymal intrahippocampal veins; 10 = sulcal intrahippocampal veins; 11 = subiculum veins.

addition to its uncal branch, the anterior choroidal artery also leads to hippocampal branches on its way to the choroidal plexuses of the temporal horn [6–8]. The superficial hippocampal arteries most frequently arise from the trunk of the posterior cerebral artery, from its choroidal posterolateral, splenial, inferior, temporal branches, and from the anterior choroidal artery. It is rare that the arteries arise predominantly from the anterior choroidal artery [9, 10].

Of the superficial hippocampal arteries, the most developed and frequently present are the medial hippocampal arteries. The posterior hippocampal arteries often follow alongside them on the surface of the subiculum and vascularize the cortex in this area. Approaching the margo denticulatus, they follow a longitudinal path, with numerous anastomoses, parallel to the hippocampal sulcus. The perforating arteries arise from this anastomotic network and enter the hippocampus between the indentations of the margo denticulatus and vascularize the hippocampal body and tail (fig. 4) [1, 5].

The anterior hippocampal artery partly forms the dense hippocampo-parahippocampal arterial complex at the uncal apex. It penetrates the uncal sulcus and reappears on the cortical surface to vascularize the entorhinal area. In the uncal sulcus, it forms branches that penetrate between the digitationes of the hippocampal head to ensure vascularization. The uncal branch of the anterior choroidal artery frequently anastomoses with the anterior hippocampal artery deep inside the uncal sulcus and thus also contributes to the vascularization of the hippocampal head [1, 5].

Deep Hippocampal Arteries

Knowledge of the location of the intrahippocampal vessels stems from the work of Duvernoy [1]. The superficial hippocampal arteries give rise to intraparenchymal arteries which can be classified into the large ventral intrahippocampal arteries, large dorsal intrahippocampal arteries, small ventral intrahippocampal arteries, and small dorsal intrahippocampal arteries (fig. 4).

The large ventral intrahippocampal arteries penetrate the hippocampus between the teeth of the margo denticulatus and then vascularize CA1 and CA2. The large dorsal intrahippocampal arteries have a shorter path, passing between the teeth of the margo denticulatus and entering CA4 and CA3. They also vascularize the distal part of the gyrus dentatus via rectilinear arteries.

The small ventral intrahippocampal arteries enter the surface of the margo denticulatus and vascularize the proximal part of the gyrus dentatus. The small dorsal intrahippocampal arteries cross the surface of the margo denticulatus, then enter the fimbriodentate sulcus and vascularize CA3 and a small part of CA4.

Venous Vascularization of the Hippocampus

Venous vascularization of the hippocampus is provided by the intrahippocampal veins, comprising the subependymal intrahippocampal veins and sulcal intrahippocampal veins, which drain into the superficial hippocampal veins [1].

The superficial hippocampal veins form two venous arches: the venous arch of the fimbriodentate sulcus and the venous arch of the hippocampal sulcus, located in the corresponding sulci. Both venous arches drain into the basal vein anteriorly by the inferior ventricular vein, and posteriorly by the medial atrial vein. The basal vein is a satellite of the posterior cerebral artery on the lateral surface of the mesencephalon in the ambient cistern, and drains posteriorly into the vein of Galen [11, 12].

The venous arch of the fimbriodentate sulcus receives the subependymal intrahippocampal veins, visible at the alveus on the surface of the intraventricular part of the hippocampus. The venous arch of the hippocampal sulcus receives the sulcal intrahippocampal veins that arise from the hippocampus at the junction of the gyrus dentatus and the cornu ammonis [1] (fig. 4).

References

1 Duvernoy H: The Human Hippocampus. Functional Anatomy, Vascularization and Serial Sections with MRI, ed 3. Berlin, Springer, 2005.
2 Nieuwenhuys R, Voogd J, van Huijzen C: The Human Central Nervous System. A Synopsis and Atlas, ed 4. Berlin, Springer, 2007.
3 Haegelen C, Berton E, Darnault P, Morandi X: A revised classification of the temporal branches of the posterior cerebral artery. Surg Radiol Anat 2012;34: 385–391.
4 Stephens R, Stilwell D: Arteries and veins of the human brain. Springfield, Thomas, 1969.
5 Marinkovic S, Milisavljevic M, Puskas L: Microvascular anatomy of the hippocampal formation. Surg Neurol 1992;37:339–349.
6 Rhoton AL, Fujii K, Fradd B: Microsurgical anatomy of the anterior choroidal artery. Surg Neurol 1979; 12:171–187.
7 Morandi X, Brassier G, Darnault P, Mercier P, Scarabin JM, Duval JM: Microsurgical anatomy of the anterior choroidal artery. Surg Radiol Anat 1996;18: 275–280.
8 Cosson A, Tatu L, Vuillier F, Parratte B, Diop M, Monnier G: Arterial vascularization of the human thalamus: extra-parenchymal arterial groups. Surg Radiol Anat 2003;25:408–415.
9 Erdem A, Yasargil MG, Roth P: Microsurgical anatomy of the hippocampal arteries. J Neurosurg 1993; 79:256–265.
10 Huther G, Dörfl J, van der Loos H, Jeanmonod D: Micronanatomic and vascular aspects of the temporomesial region. Neurosurgery 1998;43:1118–1136.
11 Duvernoy H: The Superficial Veins of the Human Brain. Berlin, Springer, 1975.
12 Huang Y, Wolf B: The basal cerebral vein and its tributaries; in Newton T, Potts D (eds): Radiology of the Skull and Brain. St. Louis, Mosby, 1974, pp 2111–2154.

Professor Laurent Tatu
Department of Neuromuscular diseases, CHU Jean-Minjoz
Boulevard Fleming
FR–25030 Besançon Cedex (France)
E-Mail laurent.tatu@univ-fcomte.fr

Szabo K, Hennerici MG (eds): The Hippocampus in Clinical Neuroscience.
Front Neurol Neurosci. Basel, Karger, 2014, vol 34, pp 26–35 (DOI: 10.1159/000357026)

Coordinated Network Activity in the Hippocampus

Andreas Draguhn · Martin Keller · Susanne Reichinnek

University of Heidelberg, Institute for Physiology and Pathophysiology, Heidelberg, Germany

Abstract

The hippocampus expresses a variety of highly organized network states which bind its individual neurons into collective modes of activity. These patterns go along with characteristic oscillations of extracellular potential known as theta, gamma, and ripple oscillations. Such network oscillations share some important features throughout the entire central nervous system of higher animals: they are restricted to a defined behavioral state, they are mostly generated by subthreshold synaptic activity, and they entrain active neurons to fire action potentials at strictly defined phases of the oscillation cycle, thereby providing a unifying 'zeitgeber' for coordinated multineuronal activity. Recent work from the hippocampus of rodents and humans has revealed how the resulting spatiotemporal patterns support the formation of neuronal assemblies which, in our present understanding, form the neuronal correlate of spatial, declarative, or episodic memories. In this review, we introduce the major types of spatiotemporal activity patterns in the hippocampus, describe the underlying neuronal mechanisms, and illustrate the concept of memory formation within oscillating networks. Research on hippocampus-dependent memory has become a key model system at the interface between cellular and cognitive neurosciences. The next step will be to translate our increasing insight into the mechanisms and systemic functions of neuronal networks into urgently needed new therapeutic strategies.

Since the early days of electroencephalography it has been clear that the brain expresses highly organized patterns of electrical activity [1]. These patterns represent mostly oscillations, i.e. rhythmic alterations of electrical potentials which can be easily recorded from the scalp but are also present in deeper nuclei of the brain. These patterns occur in a large variety of different waveforms, amplitudes, frequencies, and spatial distributions, and the electrical state of the brain changes rapidly depending on vigilance and the behavioral or cognitive state of the human being or animal. As an early example, Berger [1] described the 'alpha-blockade', a sudden disappearance of occipital alpha rhythms when the subject opens his/her eyes or starts mental operations like mathematical calculations.

Why is brain activity organized in rhythms? Cumulative evidence from the past two decades provides interesting answers to this question, and a good part of these theories is derived from studies of the human and rodent hippocampus. Before going into any detail we shall briefly summarize key features of oscillating brain activity:

- Oscillations are state-dependent. Any change of behavior or vigilance goes along with characteristic changes in oscillation patterns. This is particularly obvious during sleep, where the frequency of EEG oscillations is the major diagnostic tool for sleep staging.
- Oscillations synchronize neurons within local networks. Almost every single neuron within an oscillating network undergoes synchronous membrane potential fluctuations. As a result, neurons are activated in highly organized spatial and temporal patterns.
- Oscillations couple different brain areas. Rhythmic patterns can occur in a coherent (sometimes even synchronous) manner between distant networks, resulting in transient functional coupling of neuronal activity.
- Pyramidal neurons fire action potentials sparsely during network oscillations. Macroscopic rhythms (like the EEG) are therefore mostly generated by summed synaptic potentials rather than by action potentials. At the level of single neurons, network oscillations cause mostly subthreshold synaptic potentials.

The above-mentioned features of network oscillations support one (of several possible) conceptual framework emphasizing their role in cognitive processes: network oscillations provide a common timeframe for neuronal activity, or more simply, they represent a clock [2, 3]. Imagine that all neurons within a local network experience synchronous synaptic inputs. As a consequence, they will follow the same cycles of depolarization (excitation) and hyperpolarization (the simplest form of synaptic inhibition). Their probability to fire action potentials follows the same temporal pattern such that discharges – even if rare for individual neurons – will occur at a well-defined phase of the oscillation cycle. Thus, the global network oscillation gives rise to a highly organized pattern of spatially and temporally distributed action potentials. Such emerging multicellular spike patterns are believed to underlie behavioral or cognitive operations of the nervous system, e.g. the formation of percepts, motor actions, or memories [4]. Within this concept, the hippocampus has become one of the most extensively studied brain regions. At present, much of our conceptual framework on spatiotemporal activity patterns comes from this model system in rodents and humans.

Oscillations in the Hippocampus

The neuropsychological consequences of circumscribed hippocampal lesions suggest an important role of this network for spatial, episodic, and declarative memory formation [5]. Among these functions, spatial memory can be easily studied in rodents. Correlative behavioral and electrophysiological experiments on spatial memory formation in mice and rats have become a highly important model system in cognitive neurosciences. Not surprisingly, network oscillations play a key role in these considerations.

To explain possible cellular and network concepts of oscillations and spatial memory formation, we will first outline the basic properties of memory-related hippocampal activity patterns. Then, we will address the underlying cellular mechanisms. Finally, we will give some examples for the different roles of hippocampal subfields and connected brain regions, putting the concept into a more systemic context.

Basic Properties of Memory-Related Activity Patterns

Mechanistic insight into the cellular organization of spatial memory began with the discovery of place cells by John O'Keefe and Jonathan Dostrovski in 1971 [6, 7]. Using extracellular depth electrodes in the hippocampus of freely moving rats, they recorded single-unit activity which corresponded to action potentials of individual neurons. O'Keefe and Dostrovski found that single hippocampal units (i.e. neurons) were only activated when the animal was at a circumscribed place (place field) within its local environment. When the rat visited other locations, they kept silent. Accordingly, they termed these neurons 'place cells'.

While the mechanisms underlying selective activation of place cells are not completely known, it is likely that they receive convergent synaptic input from the entorhinal cortex. This area, in turn, receives polymodal sensory information from many different brain regions. In this way, the hippocampus is 'instructed' about the context (spatial, visual, olfactory, haptic, and acoustic properties) of an animal's environment. The hippocampus itself seems to transform this context-dependent information into lasting changes of activity, such that spatial memories can be formed. This process occurs within highly ordered temporal activity patterns. During exploration of its territory, the rat's hippocampus expresses a prominent theta rhythm (5–10 Hz in rodents) and the place-dependent action potential firing of place cells is entrained by this network oscillation (fig. 1a). When the animal enters the place field of a given cell, it will discharge at a late phase of the theta cycle. Subsequently, while the animal proceeds through the respective field, firing will shift to ever earlier phases of the theta cycle. This systematic shift between the firing phase and network oscillation is called phase precession [8]. While the animal crosses a certain place field, place cells of neighboring overlapping fields may already start firing. This will again begin at a late phase of the theta cycle before moving to earlier phases. As a result, cells of 'later' place fields fire with a temporal delay towards cells from preceding place fields. Applying this mechanism to multiple place fields will then automatically generate sequences of place cell activity. In other words: place cell sequences form a representation of the animal's route through its environment. These temporal relationships are organized by theta activity in the hippocampal network. More detailed studies have revealed that the theta oscillation is superimposed by a second, faster network rhythm called gamma oscillation (30–100 Hz).

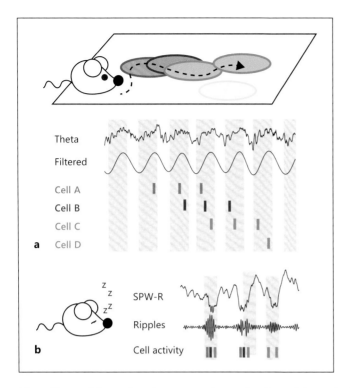

Fig. 1. Place cell formation, theta precession, and replay. **a** Schematic view of a rodent passing through different place fields (colored areas). As the mouse enters a receptive field of a given place cell (cells A–D), the specific cell starts spiking (colored ticks). Proceeding through the receptive field of a cell shifts activity from the peak of the underlying theta oscillation (raw data and 4- to 12-Hz-filtered trace) to the preceding phase of the cycle (phase precession). This process results in a temporal sequence of place cell activity which represents the trajectory of the mouse. **b** During sleep or awake immobility place cell sequences are reactivated on top of sharp-wave ripple oscillations (replay). These oscillations consist of a slow wave superimposed by a high-frequency oscillation (see raw data and 120- to 250-Hz-filtered trace).

The interaction between two rhythmic activity patterns has inspired models about the mnestic capacity of single theta phases [3] and seems to vary depending on cognitive tasks. Thus, 'meaningful' sequences of cellular activity are organized by underlying global network oscillations which themselves show highly differentiated patterns.

The concept of spatial memory formation through temporal sequences of place cells experienced an important extension when Mathew Wilson Skaggs and Bruce McNaughton [9] found that such sequences of place cell firing were reactivated during subsequent inactive phases. Their initial observation and subsequent investigations revealed that such replay of formerly established place cell sequences occurs in states of awake immobility or slow-wave sleep (fig. 1b). At the network level, this pattern is organized by a completely different activity pattern termed sharp-wave ripple complexes (SPW-R). Sharp-wave ripples are generated in the CA3 subfield of the hippocampus and travel along the hippocampal output loop into the entorhinal cortex.

This activity provides a 'readout' signal which has been suggested to transfer previously stored spatial information into neocortical networks [10]. In conclusion, two different types of network oscillation serve as organizing principles of meaningful multineuronal activity patterns in two different states.

Spatial Memory Formation within Different Network Oscillations

The discovery of replay by Skaggs and McNaughton provides evidence for an earlier proposed model: the two-stage model of spatial memory formation [11]. During active exploration, sequential activation of place cells forms a representation of space – this activity is accompanied by theta and gamma oscillations. Subsequently, the same sequences are replayed during the distinct pattern of SPW-R which transfers the information into the neocortex for long-term storage. Supporting evidence comes from patients with hippocampal lesions. Damage to both hippocampi causes anterograde amnesia of hippocampus-dependent contents, i.e. spatial, declarative, or episodic contents. In contrast, patients can still reactivate contents which had been learned prior to the pathological event. Similar deficits have been found in animals, using spatial memory as a proxy to the more differentiated neuropsychological tests in humans. In line with the postulated role of the neocortex for memory consolidation, there is also evidence for hippocampal-neocortical crosstalk during SPW-R: prefrontal areas express sleep spindles shortly after hippocampal SPW-R. A causal, rather than correlative role for SPW-R for memory consolidation has been shown by selective suppression of this pattern which did indeed impair spatial memory performance [12]. The mechanisms, however, which translate repetitive activation of hippocampal place cell sequences into lasting memories in neocortical networks remain elusive.

The evidence presented above indicates that stable activity patterns are formed during theta oscillations. This implies that the theta state of hippocampal networks supports neuronal plasticity. Indeed, lasting changes in synaptic coupling states are easily induced by activation of synaptic inputs at theta frequency. This may be linked to the main neuromodulator which induces the theta-gamma state, acetylcholine. Hippocampal networks receive intense long-range cholinergic input from septal nuclei which may support plasticity during active wakefulness. Thus, oscillation patterns and concentrations of neuromodulators may synergistically support the formation of memory-encoding multineuronal ensembles in the hippocampus.

Cellular Mechanisms of Hippocampal Oscillations

A prominent common mechanism of almost all oscillations is the dominant role of inhibitory interneurons. In higher brain regions, these neurons are GABAergic and activate GABA-gated chloride channels ($GABA_A$ receptors) in their postsynaptic target cells. This will usually lower the probability of action potential generation by membrane hyperpolarization or electrical shunting, depending on chloride equilibrium [13]. Importantly, inhibitory postsynaptic potentials follow a characteristic time course, defined by the rapid onset and slower decay time course of $GABA_A$ receptor activation. The activity of interneurons sets the spatial-temporal conditions for different network oscillations either by local connections or long-range projections from other brain regions.

A simplified model of an inhibition-dependent network oscillation is based on feedback inhibitory interneurons, a prominent element of almost all neuronal circuits (fig. 2a). Such interneurons receive input from axon collaterals of local excitatory cells, and they project back onto the same cells. This negative feedback circuit guarantees that overall activity is maintained within a physiological range, avoiding hyperactivity or complete silence. Recent evidence, however, shows that the same mechanism is also suited to generate network oscillations [14]. Feedback interneurons typically have a widespread axonal plexus innervating hundreds or thousands of local target cells. They are also mutually connected both by GABAergic axon terminals and gap junctions (electrical synapses) which favor synchronization of their activity.

Taken together, these properties are sufficient to generate a local network oscillation. Active excitatory principal cells will activate feedback interneurons. These interneurons synchronize their activity and generate a strong inhibitory output to most, if not all, local pyramidal cells. The resulting inhibitory postsynaptic potential will silence the main cell population before it decays and excitability increases again, such that a new cycle of activity can start (fig. 2b). Therefore, such feedback circuits can generate cyclic patterns of activity with a time constant in the order of magnitude of the IPSP duration which is the time-limiting step in this process [15]. For example, an IPSP duration of 25 ms will result in an oscillatory frequency of approximately 40 Hz, corresponding to classical hippocampal gamma oscillations. Of course, this simplified scenario has gained numerous extensions and specifications for different brain regions and oscillation patterns [16].

Switches between Different Oscillation Patterns

How does a hard-wired network like the hippocampus then support switches between different network oscillations? While this question is not entirely solved, two important mechanisms have been identified: interneuron heterogeneity and the effects of neuromodulators. The latter has already been mentioned above: different behavioral or cognitive states go along with different activity of neuromodulatory systems such as the cholinergic, adrenergic, serotonergic, and others. For example, gamma oscillations can be induced by cholinergic activity, similar to certain forms of hippocampal theta oscillations [17]. Extending this concept, recent work has revealed

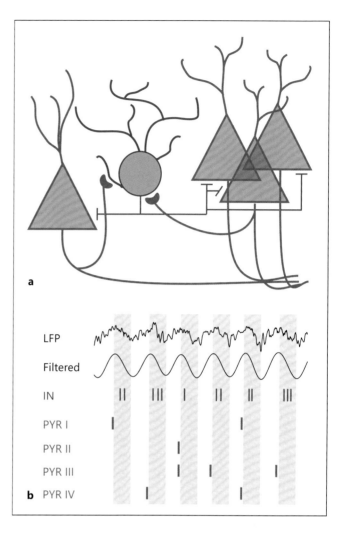

Fig. 2. Generation of oscillating activity by interactions between interneurons and pyramidal cells. **a** The scheme shows pyramidal cells (blue) and a GABAergic interneuron (red). Note that the interneuron receives input from axon collaterals of pyramidal cells. When the interneuron is depolarized above threshold it will fire an action potential and inhibit the population of local pyramidal cells (feedback inhibition). **b** Typically, pyramidal cells (blue ticks) show sparse spiking whereas interneurons fire frequently during each oscillation cycle. As a result, pyramidal cells can form multiple different functional assemblies while the global oscillatory activity is formed by subthreshold excitation and inhibition in all neurons of the network.

multiple subtypes of interneurons with specific and different functions. Defined interneurons support certain patterns of network activity, and they control different portions of principal cells, e.g. certain dendritic segments with specific synaptic input sites or the somatic and axonal region where action potentials are generated [18]. Within the CA1 subfield of the hippocampus, more than 20 different types of interneurons have been described. Each of these cell types expresses a peculiar pattern of afferent and efferent connectivity, receptor profile, synaptic dynamics, cotransmitters, and other molecular and structural properties. Recordings from single cells in living animals has confirmed that different types of neurons are selectively activated during different network states. Thus, neuronal diversity serves as an important mechanism underlying the state-dependent switching between different oscillatory regimes.

Lastly, it should be mentioned that electrical coupling between neurons might be more important for organizing network activity than hitherto thought. This does not only apply to inhibitory interneurons, but also to principal (excitatory) projection cells which appear to be coupled between their axons [19]. Thereby, the electrical activity of axons may be much more complex and independent from somatodendritic synaptic integration than usually described [20]. In electrically coupled axons, spikes can rapidly 'jump' from one axon to a coupled fiber, such that groups of selected axons fire synchronously independent from dendritic input. Other recent work indicates that axo-axonal coupling supports ultrarapid communication and synchronization within hippocampal networks. In addition, this mechanism would allow repetitive activation of neuronal ensembles independent from incoming environmental information.

Coordination between Hippocampal Subfields and Other Brain Regions

On a larger scale, activity is also coordinated between different hippocampal subfields and between the hippocampus and other brain regions. The hippocampal formation comprises a group of interconnected networks with intense connections to limbic nuclei (e.g. the amygdala), neocortical structures (e.g. the entorhinal and prefrontal cortices), and multiple further areas like septal nuclei and the hypothalamus. This connectivity reflects functional roles in many systems far beyond declarative, episodic, and spatial memory formation. These additional functions may be clinically relevant, e.g. with respect to stress responses; strong or chronic stressors can lead to structural damage of hippocampal neurons which may, in turn, affect connected brain regions [21, 22]. Moreover, the hippocampus plays an important role in temporal lobe epilepsy, possibly supported by its intense recurrent excitatory loops and by its marked synaptic plasticity which may underlie progressive epileptogenesis.

Each hippocampal subfield has its peculiar intrinsic properties and extrinsic connectivity, resulting in specific neuronal activity patterns. We will briefly illustrate prominent examples of the dentate gyrus, CA3, and CA1, notwithstanding that CA2, the hilar region, the subiculum and adjacent of the entorhinal, perirhinal, and parahippocampal cortices are equally important.

The dentate gyrus is a major input network, receiving multiple afferents from the entorhinal cortex via the perforant path. The most prevalent cell type in this area is the excitatory granule cell, which is characterized by small somata, high input resistance, and very negative membrane potential. In addition, the somata of dentate granule cells are strongly innervated by GABAergic synapses from inhibitory basket cells. As a consequence, they rarely reach threshold and fire very sparsely. On the other hand, their number is extremely high so that specific entorhinal input patterns excite very small specific subpopulations of granule cells. This sparse and highly distinct firing mode corresponds with the systemic property of pattern separation: slight modifications of a rat's environment result in detectable changes of the activated neuronal ensembles in the dentate gyrus [23]. Therefore, this region thus seems to be sensitive to spatial variance, rather than to the detection of similarities.

In strong contrast, the target region of the dentate granule cells, CA3, contains approximately 10 times less neurons which receive highly convergent input from granule cell axons (mossy fibers). In addition, pyramidal cells within CA3 are highly interconnected by recurrent excitatory synapses. Thus, different ensembles of dentate granule cells may converge on overlapping groups of CA3 neurons. These groups, even if incompletely activated, converge onto stable and reproducible activity patterns due to the intense recurrent excitatory connections. Behaviorally, this may correspond to pattern completion, i.e. the repetitive activation of a known network pattern even upon incomplete or slightly varied input. In the experiments described above, the pattern of units within CA3 did indeed stay constant during gradual changes in the spatial environment, but suddenly changed into a different pattern when a critical degree of change was reached [24]. Together with the plastic properties of synapses, the autoassociative network of CA3 may thus serve to form stable memories which can be easily reactivated.

CA1, finally, forms the target region of axons from CA3, called Schaffer collaterals. At the same time, CA1 (and CA2) receives input from the direct temporoammonic tract of the entorhinal cortex, such that two major pathways converge on CA1 neurons. Accordingly, CA1 has been suggested to serve a role in comparing actual information about the external world (direct input) with stored patterns resulting from previous experiences (input from CA3) [25]. Interestingly, different frequencies of gamma oscillations seem to route the flow of information in CA1 [26]. Spatially distributed neurons are transiently linked by a synchronized phased-locked gamma oscillation to either the input from CA3 or the entorhinal cortex. This is supported by previous studies reporting that inputs from these two regions arrive at different phases of the theta cycle, thereby providing different time frames for memory formation, memory consolidation, and memory retrieval.

This brief overview shall suffice to exemplify the different structure and spatiotemporal dynamics of hippocampal subfields. Additional research is needed to correlate the internal structure and external connections of each region with its contribution to cognitive and behavioral capabilities. It is also time to strengthen the causal analysis of relationships between molecular, cellular, network-level, and cognitive functions. It appears safe, however, to say that the selective and coordinated activation of neurons within oscillating networks forms an important neuronal correlate of cognitive and behavioral neuronal functions. The next challenge is to translate the growing insight from network-level memory research into new therapeutic strategies which are urgently needed for clinical treatment of amnesia and dementia.

References

1 Berger H: Über das Elektrenkephalogramm des Menschen. Arch Psychiatr 1929;87:527–570.
2 Buzsáki G, Draguhn A: Neuronal oscillations in cortical networks. Science 2004;304:1926–1929.
3 Lisman J: The theta/gamma discrete phase code occuring during the hippocampal phase precession may be a more general brain coding scheme. Hippocampus 2005;15:913–922.
4 Singer W: Neuronal synchrony: a versatile code for the definition of relations? Neuron 1999;24:49–65, 111–125.
5 Scoville WB, Milner B: Loss of recent memory after bilateral hippocampal lesions. 1957. J Neuropsychiatry Clin Neurosci 2000;12:103–113.
6 O'Keefe J, Dostrovsky J: The hippocampus as a spatial map. Preliminary evidence from unit activity in the freely-moving rat. Brain Res 1971;34:171–175.
7 O'Keefe J: Place units in the hippocampus of the freely moving rat. Exp Neurol 1976;51:78–109.
8 O'Keefe J, Recce ML: Phase relationship between hippocampal place units and the EEG theta rhythm. Hippocampus 1993;3:317–330.
9 Skaggs WE, McNaughton BL: Replay of neuronal firing sequences in rat hippocampus during sleep following spatial experience. Science 1996;271:1870–1873.
10 Ylinen A, Bragin A, Nádasdy Z, Jandó G, Szabó I, Sik A, Buzsáki G: Sharp wave-associated high-frequency oscillation (200 Hz) in the intact hippocampus: network and intracellular mechanisms. J Neurosci 1995; 15:30–46.
11 Buzsaki G: Two-stage model of memory trace formation: a role for 'noisy' brain states. Neuroscience 1989;31:551–570.
12 Girardeau G, Benchenane K, Wiener SI, Buzsáki G, Zugaro MB: Selective suppression of hippocampal ripples impairs spatial memory. Nat Neurosci 2009; 12:1222–1223.
13 Blaesse P, Airaksinen MS, Rivera C, Kaila K: Cation-chloride cotransporters and neuronal function. Neuron 200;61:820–838.
14 Möhler H: Molecular regulation of cognitive functions and developmental plasticity: impact of GABAA receptors. J Neurochem 2007;102:1–12.
15 Traub RD, Whittington MA, Colling SB, Buzsáki G, Jefferys JG: Analysis of gamma rhythms in the rat hippocampus in vitro and in vivo. J Physiol 1996; 493:471–484.
16 Whittington MA, Cunningham MO, LeBeau FE, Racca C, Traub RD: Multiple origins of the cortical γ rhythm. Dev Neurobiol 2011;71:92–106.
17 Cobb SR, Buhl EH, Halasy K, Paulsen O, Somogyi P: Synchronization of neuronal activity in hippocampus by individual GABAergic interneurons. Nature 1995;378:75–78.
18 Klausberger T, Somogyi P: Neuronal diversity and temporal dynamics: the unity of hippocampal circuit operations. Science 2008;321:53–57.
19 Traub RD, Bibbig A, LeBeau FE, Buhl EH, Whittington MA: Cellular mechanisms of neuronal population oscillations in the hippocampus in vitro. Annu Rev Neurosci 2004;27:247–278.
20 Bähner F, Weiss EK, Birke G, Maier N, Schmitz D, Rudolph U, Frotscher M, Traub RD, Both M, Draguhn A: Cellular correlate of assembly formation in oscillating hippocampal networks in vitro. Proc Natl Acad Sci USA 2011;108:E607–E616.
21 Stankiewicz AM, Swiergiel AH, Lisowski P: Brain epigenetics of stress adaptations in the brain. Brain Res Bull 2013;98:76–92.
22 Krugers HJ, Karst H, Joels M: Interactions between noradrenaline and corticosteroids in the brain: from electrical activity to cognitive performance. Front Cell Neurosci 2012;6:15.
23 Gothard KM, Hoffman KL, Battaglia FP, McNaughton BL: Dentate gyrus and CA1 ensemble activity during spatial reference frame shifts in the presence and absence of visual input. J Neurosci 2001;21: 7284–7292.
24 Leutgeb S, Leutgeb JK, Treves A, Moser MB, Moser E: Distinct ensemble codes in hippocampal areas CA3 and CA1. Science 2004;305:1295–1298.
25 Vinogradova OS: Hippocampus as comparator: role of the two input and two output systems of the hippocampus in selection and registration of information. Hippocampus 2001;11:578–598.
26 Colgin LL, Denninger T, Fyhn M, Hafting T, Bonnevie T, Jensen O, Moser MB, Moser EI: Frequency of gamma oscillations routes flow of information in the hippocampus. Nature 2009;462:353–357.

Prof. Dr. Andreas Draguhn
Institut für Physiologie und Pathophysiologie, Universität Heidelberg
Im Neuenheimer Feld 326
DE–69120 Heidelberg (Germany)
E-Mail andreas.draguhn@physiologie.uni-heidelberg.de

Szabo K, Hennerici MG (eds): The Hippocampus in Clinical Neuroscience.
Front Neurol Neurosci. Basel, Karger, 2014, vol 34, pp 36–50 (DOI: 10.1159/000356418)

What Animals Can Teach Clinicians about the Hippocampus

Pierre Lavenex[a, b] · Pamela Banta Lavenex[a] · Grégoire Favre[b]

[a]Laboratory for Experimental Research on Behavior, Institute of Psychology, University of Lausanne, Lausanne, and [b]Laboratory of Brain and Cognitive Development, Fribourg Center for Cognition, University of Fribourg, Fribourg, Switzerland

Abstract

Abnormalities in hippocampal structure and function have been reported in a number of human neuropathological and neurodevelopmental disorders, including Alzheimer's disease, autism spectrum disorders, Down syndrome, epilepsy, and schizophrenia. Given the complexity of these disorders, animal studies are invaluable and remain to date irreplaceable, providing fundamental knowledge regarding the basic mechanisms underlying normal and pathological human brain structure and function. However, there is a prominent ill-conceived view in current research that scientists should be restricted to using animal models of human diseases that can lead to results applicable to humans within a few years. Although there is no doubt that translational studies of this kind are important and necessary, limiting animal studies to applicable questions is counterproductive and will ultimately lead to a lack of knowledge and an inability to address human health problems. Here, we discuss findings regarding the normal postnatal development of the monkey hippocampal formation, which provide an essential framework to consider the etiologies of different neuropathological disorders affecting human hippocampal structure and function. We focus on studies of gene expression in distinct hippocampal regions that shed light on some basic mechanisms that might contribute to the etiology of schizophrenia. We argue that researchers, as well as clinicians, should not consider the use of animals in research only as 'animal models' of human diseases, as they will continue to need and benefit from a better understanding of the normal structure and functions of the hippocampus in 'model animals'.

© 2014 S. Karger AG, Basel

Experimental studies conducted with animals are invaluable and remain to date irreplaceable, providing some of the fundamental knowledge regarding the basic mechanisms underlying normal and pathological human physiology. The study of the brain, and the hippocampus in particular, is no exception and most of the information regarding the basic structure and functions of the hippocampal formation have derived from animal studies [1]. Over the years, however, a gradual shift has occurred in the type of scientific studies performed with animals, going from descriptive studies of the organization of the nervous system, to experimental studies of normal brain function, to animal models of human disease.

Currently, a prominent ill-conceived view of which research with animals should be encouraged, funded, or even allowed posits that scientists should be restricted to only using animal models of human diseases that can lead to results applicable to humans within a few years. Although there is no doubt that translational studies of this kind are important and necessary, limiting animal studies to currently applicable questions is counterproductive and will ultimately lead to a lack of knowledge and an inability to address human health problems. Moreover, defining what is dispensable in science and foreseeing which experiment will lead to truly applicable results are very difficult and often likely to be wrong. Failure is part of the scientific endeavor and should be embraced, as much as success, as long as we have a chance to gain new knowledge by performing an experiment or making an observation.

A perfect example of this is the discovery of penicillin by Sir Alexander Fleming in 1928. It was a failed experiment, the accidental contamination of a bacteria culture plate by a mold, that led to the isolation and identification of this widely-used antibacterial substance. In his Nobel Prize acceptance speech in 1945, Fleming declared:

> We all know that chance, fortune, fate or destiny – call it what you will has played a considerable part in many of the great discoveries in science. We do not know how many, for all scientists who have hit on something new have not disclosed exactly how it happened. We do know, though, that in many cases it was a chance observation which took them into a track which eventually led to a real advance in knowledge or practice. This is especially true of the biological sciences for there we are dealing with living mechanisms about which there are enormous gaps in our knowledge.

Many scientists, including a number of other Nobel laureates, have shared his view. Furthermore to date, there are still enormous gaps in our knowledge of normal brain structure and functions.

Here, we very humbly discuss the continuous need to obtain fundamental information regarding how the normal brain is built and works. We argue that researchers, as well as clinicians, should not consider the use of animals in research only as 'animal models' of human diseases since science, and medicine in particular, will continue to need and indeed will benefit greatly from a better understanding of the structure and function of biological systems in various organisms or 'model animals'. Given the focus of this book on the hippocampus, we consider specific examples illustrating how fundamental knowledge of the normal patterns of postnatal development of the monkey hippocampal formation can shed light on the etiologies of human diseases affecting hippocampal structure and function.

The Primate Hippocampus: Structure

The terms 'hippocampus' and 'hippocampal formation' are often used interchangeably, yet they refer to and include different brain structures depending on the context in which they are used. Here, we do not provide an exhaustive and detailed description of the structural characteristics of the hippocampus, as this has already been done [2–4]. We use the definition of the hippocampal formation as a group of cortical regions located in the medial temporal lobe that includes the dentate gyrus, hippocampus (CA3, CA2, CA1), subiculum, presubiculum, parasubiculum, and entorhinal cortex (fig. 1). Each of these structures contains a number of different cell types and different sets of intrinsic connections, as well as interconnections with other brain regions, both of which exhibit clear and distinct topographical distributions. Altogether, these interconnected structures form a functional brain system essential for memory, which is particularly sensitive to a number of pathologies [4].

As mentioned above, most of the information regarding the structural organization of functional hippocampal circuits is derived from experimental work performed with animals, in particular rodents but also monkeys. Similarly, animal models are typically used to study the molecular and cellular basis of pathologies affecting human hippocampal structure and function. Consequently, it is important to be aware of the similarities and differences between species in order to extrapolate from the findings of fundamental research in animals to clinical problems in humans [4].

For example, let us consider that an experimental study in rats reveals that the commissural projections, which originate in the polymorphic layer of the dentate gyrus and are prominent throughout the entire septotemporal (long) axis of the rat dentate gyrus, play an important role in the generation or spread of epileptic seizures throughout the hippocampal network. These findings will be very difficult to extrapolate to humans and are very unlikely to have any direct clinical impact since the commissural projections of the primate (including humans) dentate gyrus are extremely limited and originate only from its most rostral (or uncal) portion. Rats are not monkeys, and monkeys are not humans. However, brain structures and functions that are conserved between rats and monkeys are likely to be conserved in humans. One striking example is the central role of the hippocampus in allocentric spatial learning and memory processes [5–7].

To be extremely clear, we are not arguing that experimental work aimed at understanding the fundamentals of brain structure and functions should not be performed in rodents. However, great care must be taken when extrapolating results from one species to another [8, 9]. Rhesus monkeys, with their phylogenetic proximity to humans, represent an unparalleled model in which empirical and systematic investigations of the normal and pathological development of brain-cognition interactions can be undertaken. Nonhuman primate research is thus particularly important to bridge potential gaps between experimental studies in rodents and clinical applications in humans.

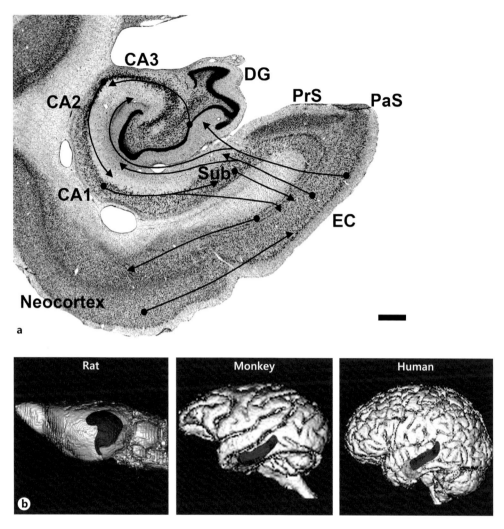

Fig. 1. a Schematic representation of the hierarchical organization of the main serial and parallel pathways through the different regions of the rhesus macaque monkey *(Macaca mulatta)* hippocampal formation. EC = Entorhinal cortex; DG = dentate gyrus; CA3, CA2, CA1 = fields of the hippocampus proper; Sub = subiculum; PrS = presubiculum; PaS = parasubiculum. Scale bar = 1 mm. **b** Volume-rendered MRI of rat, monkey, and human brains illustrating the relative positions of the dentate gyrus + hippocampus + subiculum (in red) and the entorhinal cortex (in green). MRI of the rat brain, courtesy of Dr. G. Allan Johnson, Center for In Vivo Microscopy, Duke University, NIH/NCRR National Resource (P41 05959).

The Primate Hippocampus: Development

Understanding the normal development of the hippocampal formation can provide invaluable information about its functions and its susceptibility to pathologies across the lifespan [4, 7]. Until recently, there was little information on the structural development of the different regions of the primate hippocampal formation and the impact of their maturation on the emergence of particular functions [7]. For example, in the case of developmental amnesia, patients who sustained hippocampal damage early in life exhibit memory impairments affecting preferentially episodic memory (the memory for autobiographical events), whereas semantic memory (the memory for facts about the world) is somehow preserved [10]. In contrast, a hippocampal lesion in adults generally impairs both semantic and episodic memory processes [11]. We have shown similar functional plasticity in monkeys that received hippocampal lesions early in life. Hippocampal lesions prevent spatial relational learning in adult-lesioned monkeys [5], whereas spatial relational learning persists following neonatal lesions [12]. Preliminary findings from our laboratory suggest that significant reorganization of specific brain circuits might contribute to the recovery of function following early but not late lesions [Lavenex et al., unpubl. data]. Now, we briefly discuss our findings regarding the normal postnatal development of the monkey hippocampal formation [13, 14] (fig. 2) that provide an essential framework to consider the etiologies of different neurodevelopmental disorders affecting human hippocampal structure and functions.

Neurogenesis in the Dentate Gyrus
The dentate gyrus is one of only two regions of the mammalian brain where substantial neurogenesis occurs postnatally (rats: [15], monkeys: [16], humans: [17]). In a first study [13], we demonstrated that about 40% of the total number of granule cells found in 5- to 10-year-old monkeys are added to the granule cell layer postnatally, with a peak (about 25%) in the first 3 months after birth. We also found significant levels of cell proliferation, neurogenesis, and cell death in the context of an overall stable number of granule cells in mature monkeys. The overall distribution of cell proliferation that we described in newborn monkeys was similar to that observed in newborn humans [18]. Importantly, we established that the developmental period during which a significant number of neurons are added to the monkey granule cell layer is longer than previously thought [16]. In the absence of strict quantification of human cases older than 1 year of age, our findings in monkeys suggest that sustained levels of developmental neurogenesis might continue and impact the dentate gyrus structure until at least 4 years of age in humans. Importantly, we also estimated the number of new neurons that could potentially be integrated into the granule cell layer of mature monkeys. We found that postnatal neurogenesis has a similar potential in rats and monkeys, i.e. the renewal of the entire population of granule cells during an individual's lifetime. It is therefore likely to be the case in humans as well.

Maturation of Distinct Hippocampal Circuits
In a second quantitative study of the postnatal structural development of the monkey hippocampal formation [14], we showed that distinct hippocampal regions and layers exhibit different profiles of structural development during early postnatal life

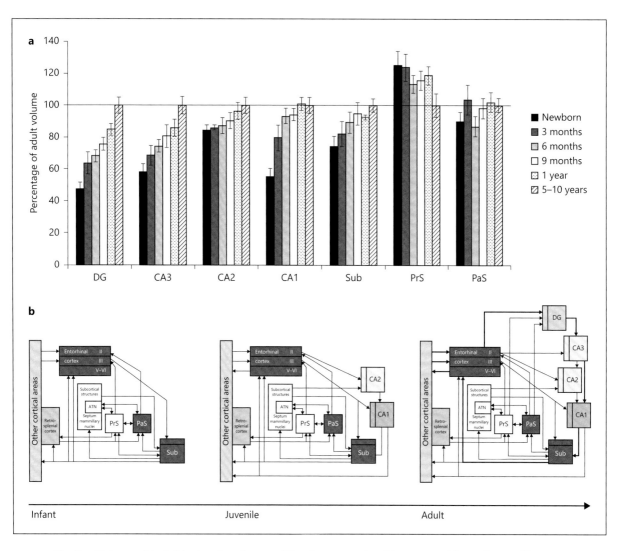

Fig. 2. a Volume of individual regions/layers of the rhesus monkey hippocampal formation at different ages during early postnatal development (expressed as percentage of the volume of the layer/region observed in 5- to 10-year-old monkeys; averages ± standard errors of the mean). **b** Hierarchical model of the postnatal maturation of the primate hippocampal formation. ATN = Anterior thalamic nuclei; DG = dentate gyrus; CA3, CA2, CA1 = fields of the hippocampus proper; Sub = subiculum; PrS = presubiculum; PaS = parasubiculum; II, III, V, VI = layers of the entorhinal cortex.

(fig. 2). Specifically, we found a protracted period of neuron addition in the dentate gyrus throughout the first postnatal year (see above), and a concomitant late maturation of the granule cell population and individual dentate gyrus layers that extended beyond the first year of life. Together with the late maturation of the granule cells, it has been reported that the mossy cells, the major targets of the granule cell projections in the polymorphic layer, exhibit clear morphological changes in soma and dendritic structure until at least 9 months of age in monkeys [19] and at least 30 months of age in humans [20]. Indeed, our analyses revealed a 25% increase in volume of the polymorphic layer between 1 year and 5–10 years of age in monkeys. Although the postnatal development of the polymorphic layer circuits is likely delayed, as compared to that of the dentate gyrus afferents reaching the molecular layer, detailed analyses of the postnatal maturation of the different cell types contained in the dentate gyrus will be necessary to provide a definite answer regarding the functional consequences of this delayed maturation. This information is particularly important to further our understanding of the etiology of temporal lobe epilepsy, as a prominent theory suggests that acquired epilepsy is an immediate network defect caused primarily by initial neuron loss during early postnatal life, most likely a loss of dentate gyrus mossy cells [21].

The development of CA3 generally parallels that of the dentate gyrus. However, the distal portion of CA3, which receives direct entorhinal cortex projections, matures earlier than the proximal portion of CA3. At the cellular level, we found that the proximal CA3 pyramidal neurons exhibit significant changes in soma size within the first 3–6 postnatal months. In contrast, the size of distal CA3 pyramidal neurons does not vary during postnatal development. Our quantitative data are thus in agreement with the qualitative report by Seress and Ribak [22] showing that the somas and dendrites of distal CA3 pyramidal neurons exhibit adult-like ultrastructural features at birth. To our knowledge, there is no published information on the ultrastructural characteristics of developing proximal CA3 pyramidal neurons.

CA1 matures relatively earlier than the dentate gyrus and CA3, despite the fact that CA3 pyramidal neurons contribute the largest projection to CA1 pyramidal neurons. Interestingly, CA1 stratum lacunosum-moleculare, in which direct entorhinal cortex projections terminate, matures earlier than CA1 strata oriens, pyramidale, and radiatum, in which the CA3 projections terminate. Our quantitative measurements are in agreement with qualitative reports of a later myelination of fibers in strata pyramidale and radiatum, as compared to stratum lacunosum-moleculare, in CA1 of humans [23].

The subiculum develops earlier than the dentate gyrus, CA3, and CA1, but not CA2. However, similar to CA1, the molecular layer of the subiculum, in which the entorhinal cortex projections terminate, is overall more mature in the first postnatal year, as compared to the stratum pyramidale in which most of the CA1 projections terminate. Unlike other hippocampal fields, volumetric measurements suggest regressive events in the structural maturation of presubicular neurons and circuits. Finally, areal and neuron soma size measurements reveal an early maturation of the parasubiculum. Two unique features of these structures, as compared to other hippocampal regions, are their reciprocal connections with the anterior thalamic nuclear complex and their heavy cholinergic innervation. Accordingly, cell circuits in the presubiculum and parasubiculum might contribute to some of the earliest functions subserved by the hippocampal formation (fig. 2). A detailed discussion of the implications of these findings with respect to the emergence of distinct 'hippocampus-dependent' memory processes in humans can be found in [24].

What Animals Can Teach Clinicians about Hypoxic Lesions and Febrile Seizures

In an effort to understand the molecular basis of the normal development of the hippocampal formation and its susceptibility to a number of different pathologies, we launched a series of experiments examining the regulation of gene expression in distinct regions of the monkey hippocampal formation during postnatal development. In a first study [25], we characterized the molecular signature of individual hippocampal regions in an attempt to understand the paradox that, although the hippocampus plays a central role in the brain network essential for memory function, it is also the brain structure that is most sensitive to hypoxic-ischemic episodes. We found that the expression of genes associated with glycolysis and glutamate metabolism in astrocytes as well as the coverage of excitatory synapses by astrocytic processes undergo significant decreases in the CA1 field of the monkey hippocampus, specifically, during postnatal development (fig. 3).

Taken together, our findings at the gene, protein, and structural levels suggest that the developmental decrease in astrocytic processes and functions may be the critical factor underlying the selective vulnerability of CA1 to hypoxic-ischemic episodes in adulthood. They also provide an explanation for the relative resistance of this brain structure to hypoxia in the perinatal period and, in particular, during the birth process. In newborns, high astrocytic coverage likely maintains sufficient glutamate reuptake to limit neuronal depolarization and excitotoxicity during mild-to-moderate hypoxic-ischemic events. In the adult, however, a lower expression level of genes associated with glycolysis or glutamate uptake and metabolism, as well as a lower astrocytic coverage of excitatory synapses in CA1, may render the system more vulnerable to a reduction in oxygen concentration.

In contrast, a major benefit that derives from decreased astrocytic coverage in adulthood is the regulation of synaptic efficacy leading to an increase in synaptic selectivity advantageous for learning. Thus, a developmental decrease of astrocytic processes and functions may therefore contribute to the emergence of adult-like selective memory function [24, 25].

Finally, the relatively high astrocytic coverage of the newborn synapses may also play a central role in the generation of febrile seizures. The highest incidence of seizures is in the first 2 years of life in humans and is most often associated with a febrile illness. Fever begins with the activation of immune response cells that produce interleukin-1, which in turn increases prostaglandin E_2 synthesis. Prostaglandins act at the level of the hypothalamus to regulate body temperature and induce fever. Interestingly, prostaglandins also stimulate calcium-dependent glutamate release in astro-

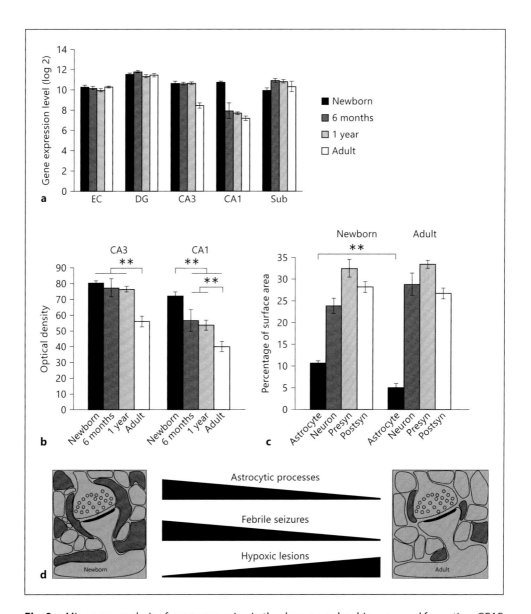

Fig. 3. a Microarray analysis of gene expression in the rhesus monkey hippocampal formation: GFAP gene expression decreased from birth to 6 months of age in CA1. GFAP gene expression decreased after 1 year of age in CA3. GFAP gene expression did not differ between CA3 and CA1 at birth, but differed at all other ages. EC = Entorhinal cortex; DG = dentate gyrus; CA3 and CA1 = fields of the hippocampus; Sub = subiculum. **b** GFAP immunostaining in the rhesus monkey hippocampus: GFAP immunostaining decreased from birth to 6 months of age in CA1. GFAP immunostaining decreased after 1 year of age in CA3. GFAP immunostaining did not differ between CA3 and CA1 at birth, but differed at all other ages. ** all p < 0.05. **c** Electron microscope evaluation of astrocytic processes around excitatory synapses in the stratum radiatum of CA1 in rhesus monkeys. The surface area occupied by astrocytic processes decreased from birth to adulthood. ** p = 0.0039. **d** Schematic representation of the changes in glial processes and putative functions from birth to adulthood, and the associated risks of exhibiting febrile seizures or suffering from hypoxic-ischemic lesions.

cytes, which can induce abnormal prolonged depolarization with repetitive spiking in CA1 pyramidal neurons leading to seizures. Thus, the relatively high astrocytic coverage of the dense network of CA1 excitatory synapses in the newborn (twice that of the adult) could explain why infants exhibit a higher incidence of febrile seizures. Conversely, the decrease in the astrocytic coverage of hippocampal excitatory synapses with development might provide the cellular basis for the decreased susceptibility to febrile seizures with age. We refer the reader to our original article [25] for a detailed discussion of the cellular mechanisms involved in these processes.

What Animals Can Teach Clinicians about Schizophrenia

Our neuroanatomical and gene expression studies described above identified different periods of postnatal development during which pathogenic factors might impact the structural and functional maturation of distinct regions of the primate hippocampal formation. The implications of our findings for autism spectrum disorders, temporal lobe epilepsy, and Down syndrome have been discussed previously [4]. Here, we focus on detailed analyses of specific patterns of gene expression and the perspectives that our findings in monkeys provide to comprehending the etiology of schizophrenia in humans [26, 27].

Pathological Findings in Humans
MRI studies consistently report reduced hippocampal volumes in first-episode schizophrenic subjects [28] and asymptomatic first-degree relatives of subjects with schizophrenia [29], indicating that hippocampal pathology is not the result of the illness or treatment, but rather contributes to the etiology of the disorder. Consistent neuropathological findings include alterations in markers of synaptic transmission for both glutamatergic and GABAergic systems [30, 31], in particular in proximal CA3 [32]. Interestingly, there are no changes in the total number of hippocampal neurons, and reports concerning neuron density or cell size differences are rather inconsistent. In contrast, there are reliable morphological changes in the dendritic and axonal arborization of dentate granule cells and the synaptic organization of CA3 pyramidal neurons. Specifically, the frequency of granule cells with basal dendrites is higher and the CA3 mossy fiber synapses are both smaller and fewer in schizophrenic patients, as compared to controls. These findings, together with the absence of obvious signs of neurodegeneration [30], suggest that schizophrenia is a neurodevelopmental disorder that might arise following the abnormal maturation of specific hippocampal circuits, namely the dendritic and axonal arborization of dentate granule cells.

As described above, our morphological data indicate that the dentate gyrus matures late, after all the other hippocampal regions. Pathogenic factors, which remain to be determined, might therefore impact the maturation of the dentate granule cells and their projections to CA3 pyramidal neurons during postnatal life. However, the absence of obvious disorganization of the dentate granule cell layer in schizophrenia suggests that pathogenic factors might act after the initial phase of postnatal developmental neurogenesis and neuron addition to the granule cell layer (i.e. a period corresponding to at least the first postnatal year in monkeys). Pathogenic factors influencing gene expression and the maturation of newly generated granule cells during late childhood or early adolescence might therefore contribute to the emergence of schizophrenic symptoms during adolescence. Accordingly, genetic predispositions to schizophrenia have been shown [30], and the identification of a number of susceptibility genes involved in postnatal neurogenesis, including DISC1, COMT, NRG1, and NPAS3, provides an additional link between the regulation of postnatal granule cell maturation and schizophrenia.

Regulation of Gene Expression in Monkeys
The hypothesis that schizophrenia emerges from the interaction between genetic predispositions and environmental factors is now widely accepted [33]. The genetic component of schizophrenia was first suspected since relatives of subjects with schizophrenia are more likely to get the illness themselves. Indeed, the risk of suffering from schizophrenia in the general population is about 1%. People who have a third-degree relative (great grandparent, first cousin) with schizophrenia are twice as likely to develop schizophrenia (2%), and those with a second-degree relative (grandparent, uncle, aunt) have an incidence varying from 2 to 6%. Finally first-degree relatives (parent, sibling) have an incidence of schizophrenia >10 times higher than the general population (13% for children, 17% for twins, 48% for identical twins). Accordingly, linkage analysis, gene expression, and genome-wide association studies have identified a number of schizophrenia susceptibility genes.

We analyzed the expression of 173 schizophrenia susceptibility genes in distinct regions of the monkey hippocampal formation during early postnatal development in order to assess the contribution of these genes to the normal development of the hippocampal formation and shed light on the pathogenesis of schizophrenia [26]. We further considered schizophrenia susceptibility genes involved in other diseases, including temporal lobe epilepsy, autism spectrum disorder, Williams syndrome, psychopathy, major depressive disorder, bipolar disorder, and Alzheimer's disease, to gain a better understanding of the possible relations between gene dysregulation, neuropathology, and clinical symptoms. We found that, as compared with all human protein-coding genes, schizophrenia susceptibility genes exhibit a differential regulation of expression in the dentate gyrus, CA3, and CA1 over the course of postnatal development (fig. 4). These findings are consistent with the hypothesis that hippocampal subfield dysfunctions could underlie psychotic manifestations in schizophrenia [34]. A number of these genes involved in synaptic transmission and dendritic morphology exhibit a developmental decrease of expression in CA3. Abnormal CA3 synaptic organization observed in schizophrenics might be related to some specific symptoms, such as loosening of association. Interestingly, changes in gene expression

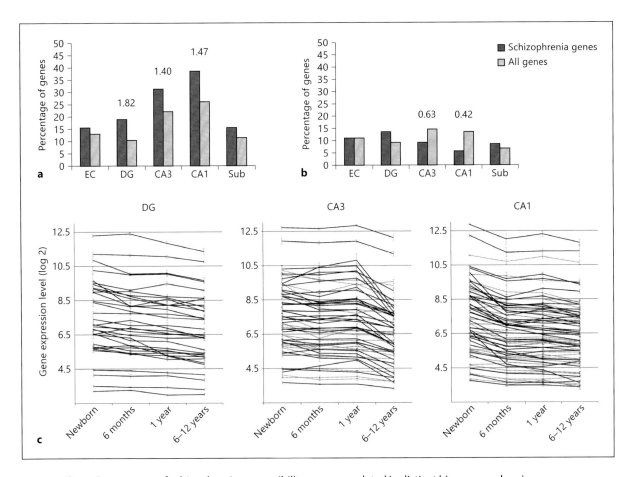

Fig. 4. Percentages of schizophrenia susceptibility genes regulated in distinct hippocampal regions from birth to adulthood: decreased expression (**a**) and increased expression (**b**). Schizophrenia susceptibility genes (173; dark gray); protein-coding human genes (20,741; light gray). DG = Dentate gyrus; EC = entorhinal cortex; Sub = subiculum. **c** Expression patterns of schizophrenia susceptibility genes regulated in the dentate gyrus, CA3 and CA1 from birth to adulthood. Dentate gyrus: 33 schizophrenia susceptibility genes exhibited lower expression levels in adult than newborn monkeys. CA3: 34 schizophrenia susceptibility genes (63%, solid lines) exhibit a significantly lower expression in adults than at any other ages. CA1: 35 schizophrenia susceptibility genes (52%, solid lines) are significantly more expressed at birth than at any other ages. Averages ± standard errors of the mean.

in CA3 might occur at a time possibly corresponding to the late appearance of the first clinical symptoms. We also found earlier changes in expression of schizophrenia susceptibility genes in CA1, which might be linked to prodromal psychotic symptoms. Finally, a number of schizophrenia susceptibility genes including APOE, BDNF, MTHFR, and SLC6A4 are involved in other disorders, and thus likely contribute to nonspecific changes in hippocampal structure and function that must be combined with the dysregulation of other genes in order to lead to schizophrenia pathogenesis.

We also used predictive bioinformatics analyses to decipher the mechanisms that underlie the coregulation of expression of hundreds of genes in different cell types at specific ages in distinct hippocampal regions [27]. Our analyses suggested that miRNAs (small RNA molecules acting as posttranscriptional regulatory elements, which have been shown to play a major role in developmental processes) may contribute to the coregulation of gene expression in different cell types (i.e. in neurons, astrocytes, oligodendrocytes) at different postnatal ages in distinct regions of the developing monkey hippocampus. Interestingly, 65% of these predicted miRNAs are conserved across species, from rodents to humans, whereas 35% are specific to primates, including humans. These miRNAs could contribute to some of the structural and functional differences observed between primate and nonprimate mammals. For example, the differences in dendritic morphology of CA1 neurons observed between rats and monkeys [8] could be related to the regulation of genes like CTNNA2 (coding for the protein alpha-N-catenin), whereas GNB5 (coding for the guanine nucleotide-binding protein, beta-5) regulation may produce differences in the electrophysiological characteristics of hippocampal neurons between these two species. Indeed, these genes were predicted to be preferentially targeted by primate-specific miRNAs and are involved, respectively, in dendritic morphology and the regulation of the stability of synaptic contacts, and in the electrophysiological properties of neurons. Other differences found among primate species might be related to the further evolution of these primate-specific miRNAs. Indeed, the numbers of miRNAs in the miR-548 and C19MC families increase from *Macaca mulatta* and *Pongo pygmaeus* to *Pan troglodytes* and *Homo sapiens*. Such species differences in miRNAs might lead to subtle differences in the regulation of gene expression that might underlie species differences in hippocampal structure and function that have emerged over the course of evolution. These differences might be particularly important to consider when extrapolating from experimental results in model animals, such as rodents and monkeys, to clinical applications in humans.

Conclusion

Experimental work performed with animals, in particular rodents but also monkeys, has provided most of our knowledge regarding the structural organization of functional hippocampal circuits. Similarly, animal models are typically used to study the molecular and cellular basis of pathologies affecting human hippocampal structure and function. It is therefore important to be aware of the similarities and differences between species (e.g. rats, monkeys, humans) in order to extrapolate from the findings of fundamental research in animals to clinical investigations in humans. Here, we discussed specific findings regarding the normal postnatal development of the monkey hippocampal formation, which provide an essential framework to consider the etiologies of different neuropathological disorders affecting human hippocampal structures and functions. We argued that researchers, as well as clinicians, should not consider the use of animals in research only as 'animal models' of human diseases, as they will continue to need and benefit from a better understanding of the normal structure and function of the hippocampus in 'model animals'.

Acknowledgements

This work was supported by grants from the Swiss National Science Foundation (PP00A-106701, PP00P3-124536) and the National Alliance for Research on Schizophrenia and Depression (NARSAD).

References

1 Amaral DG, Andersen P, Bliss T, Morris RGM, O'Keefe J: The Hippocampus Book. Oxford, Oxford University Press, 2007.

2 Amaral DG, Lavenex P: Hippocampal neuroanatomy; in Amaral DG, Andersen P, Bliss T, Morris RGM, O'Keefe J (eds): The Hippocampus Book. Oxford, Oxford University Press, 2007, pp 37–114.

3 Lavenex P: Neuroanatomic organization and fundamental functions of the hippocampus and amygdala; in Riva D, Njiokiktjien C, Bulgheroni S (eds): Brain Lesion Localization and Developmental Functions. Montrouge, John Libbey Eurotext Ltd., 2011, pp 89–118.

4 Lavenex P: Functional anatomy, development and pathology of the hippocampus; in Bartsch T (ed): Clinical Neurobiology of the Hippocampus. Oxford, University Press, 2012.

5 Banta Lavenex P, Amaral DG, Lavenex P: Hippocampal lesion prevents spatial relational learning in adult macaque monkeys. J Neurosci 2006;26:4546–4558.

6 Banta Lavenex P, Lavenex P: Spatial memory and the monkey hippocampus: not all space is created equal. Hippocampus 2009;19:8–19.

7 Lavenex P, Banta Lavenex P, Amaral DG: Postnatal development of the primate hippocampal formation. Dev Neurosci 2007;29:179–192.

8 Altemus KL, Lavenex P, Ishizuka N, Amaral DG: Morphological characteristics and electrophysiological properties of CA1 pyramidal neurons in macaque monkeys. Neuroscience 2005;136:741–756.

9 Lavenex P, Banta Lavenex P, Bennett JL, Amaral DG: Postmortem changes in the neuroanatomical characteristics of the primate brain: hippocampal formation. J Comp Neurol 2009;512:27–51.

10 Vargha-Khadem F, Gadian DG, Watkins KE, Connelly A, Van Paesschen W, Mishkin M: Differential effects of early hippocampal pathology on episodic and semantic memory. Science 1997;277:376–380.

11 Squire LR, Zola SM: Structure and function of declarative and nondeclarative memory systems. Proc Natl Acad Sci USA 1996;93:13515–13522.

12 Lavenex P, Banta Lavenex P, Amaral DG: Spatial relational learning persists following neonatal hippocampal lesions in macaque monkeys. Nat Neurosci 2007;10:234–239.

13 Jabès A, Banta Lavenex P, Amaral DG, Lavenex P: Quantitative analysis of postnatal neurogenesis and neuron number in the macaque monkey dentate gyrus. Eur J Neurosci 2010;31:273–285.

14 Jabès A, Banta Lavenex P, Amaral DG, Lavenex P: Postnatal development of the hippocampal formation: a stereological study in macaque monkeys. J Comp Neurol 2011;519:1051–1070.

15 Altman J, Das GD: Autoradiographic and histological evidence of postnatal hippocampal neurogenesis in rats. J Comp Neurol 1965;124:319–336.

16 Rakic P, Nowakowski RS: The time of origin of neurons in the hippocampal region of the rhesus monkey. J Comp Neurol 1981;196:99–128.

17 Eriksson PS, Perfilieva E, Bjork-Eriksson T, Alborn A-M, Nordborg C, Peterson DA, et al: Neurogenesis in the adult human hippocampus. Nat Med 1998;4:1313–1317.

18 Seress L: Morphological changes of the human hippocampal formation from midgestation to early childhood; in Nelson CA, Luciana M (eds): Handbook of Developmental Cognitive Neuroscience. Cambridge, MIT Press, 2001, pp 45–58.

19 Seress L, Ribak CE: Postnatal development and synaptic connections of hilar mossy cells in the hippocampal dentate gyrus of rhesus monkeys. J Comp Neurol 1995;355:93–110.

20 Seress L, Mrzljak L: Postnatal development of mossy cells in the human dentate gyrus: a light microscopic Golgi study. Hippocampus 1992;2:127–141.

21 Sloviter RS: Experimental status epilepticus in animals: what are we modeling? Epilepsia 2009; 50(suppl 12):11–13.

22 Seress L, Ribak CE: Postnatal development of CA3 pyramidal neurons and their afferents in the Ammon's horn of rhesus monkeys. Hippocampus 1995; 5:217–231.

23 Abraham H, Vincze A, Jewgenow I, Veszpremi B, Kravjak A, Gomori E, et al: Myelination in the human hippocampal formation from midgestation to adulthood. Int J Dev Neurosci 2010;28:401–410.

24 Lavenex P, Banta Lavenex P: Building hippocampal circuits to learn and remember: insights into the development of human memory. Behav Brain Res 2013;254:8–21.

25 Lavenex P, Sugden SG, Davis RR, Gregg JP, Banta Lavenex P: Developmental regulation of gene expression and astrocytic processes may explain selective hippocampal vulnerability. Hippocampus 2011; 21:142–149.

26 Favre G, Banta Lavenex P, Lavenex P: Developmental regulation of expression of schizophrenia susceptibility genes in the primate hippocampal formation. Transl Psychiatry 2012;2:e173.

27 Favre G, Banta Lavenex P, Lavenex P: miRNA regulation of gene expression: a predictive bioinformatics analysis in the postnatally developing monkey hippocampus. PLoS One 2012;7:e43435.

28 Steen RG, Mull C, McClure R, Hamer RM, Lieberman JA: Brain volume in first-episode schizophrenia: systematic review and meta-analysis of magnetic resonance imaging studies. Br J Psychiatry 2006; 188:510–518.

29 Sismanlar SG, Anik Y, Coskun A, Agaoglu B, Karakaya I, Yavuz CI: The volumetric differences of the fronto-temporal region in young offspring of schizophrenic patients. Eur Child Adolesc Psychiatry 2010; 19:151–157.

30 Harrison PJ: The hippocampus in schizophrenia: a review of the neuropathological evidence and its pathophysiological implications. Psychopharmacology (Berl) 2004;174:151–162.

31 Talbot K, Eidem WL, Tinsley CL, Benson MA, Thompson EW, Smith RJ, et al: Dysbindin-1 is reduced in intrinsic, glutamatergic terminals of the hippocampal formation in schizophrenia. J Clin Invest 2004;113:1353–1363.

32 Harrison PJ, Law AJ, Eastwood SL: Glutamate receptors and transporters in the hippocampus in schizophrenia. Ann NY Acad Sci 2003;1003:94–101.

33 Maric NP, Svrakic DM: Why schizophrenia genetics needs epigenetics: a review. Psychiatr Danub 2012; 24:2–18.

34 Tamminga CA, Stan AD, Wagner AD: The hippocampal formation in schizophrenia. Am J Psychiatry 2010;167:1178–1193.

Prof. Dr. Pierre Lavenex
Laboratory for Experimental Research on Behavior, Institute of Psychology
University of Lausanne, Géopolis 4343
CH–1015 Lausanne (Switzerland)
E-Mail pierre.lavenex@unil.ch

Szabo K, Hennerici MG (eds): The Hippocampus in Clinical Neuroscience.
Front Neurol Neurosci. Basel, Karger, 2014, vol 34, pp 51–59 (DOI: 10.1159/000356422)

Memory Function and the Hippocampus

Bertram Opitz

Department of Psychology, University of Surrey, Guildford, UK

Abstract

There has been a long tradition in memory research of adopting the view of a vital role of the medial temporal lobe and especially the hippocampus in declarative memory. Despite the broad support for this notion, there is an ongoing debate about what computations are performed by the different substructures. The present chapter summarizes several accounts of hippocampal functions in terms of the cognitive processes subserved by these structures, the information processed, and the underlying neural operations. Firstly, the value of the distinction between recollection and familiarity for the understanding of the role the hippocampus plays in memory is discussed. Then multiple lines of evidence for the role of the hippocampus in memory are considered. Cumulating evidence suggests that the hippocampus fosters the binding of disparate cortical representations of items and their spatiotemporal context into a coherent representation by means of a sparse conjunctive neural coding. This association of item and context will then lead to the phenomenological experience of recollection. In contrast, surrounding cortical areas have broader neural coding that provide a scalar signal of the similarity between two inputs (e.g. between the encoding and the retrieval). By this they form the basis of a feeling of familiarity, but also might encode the commonalities between these different inputs. However, a more complete picture of the importance of the hippocampus for declarative memories can only be drawn when the interactions of the medial temporal lobe with other brain areas are also taken into account.

© 2014 S. Karger AG, Basel

Ever since the first report of profound amnesia following medial temporal lobe (MTL) resection in patient H.M. [1], there has been a large amount of research aiming at the functional role of the MTL subregions, especially of the hippocampus, in memory. This research includes all currently available methods, including neuroimaging studies and electrophysiological recordings in humans, single cell recordings in animals, and neuropsychological studies of patients with brain injuries or of animals with experimental lesions. Although every research method has its strengths and limitations, they all converge on the view that the hippocampus operates in the service of declarative memory. One cognitive account assumes that the MTL is involved in the recognition of a previously encountered event [2–4].

Despite the broad support for this notion, there is an ongoing debate about what computations are performed by different subregions within the MTL. One prominent view capitalizing on bidirectional interconnections between the hippocampus and the surrounding MTL cortex (MTLC) proposes that the hippocampus is important for all forms of declarative memory, including recognition memory [2]. A contrasting view emphasizes the differences between the same structures within the MTL, suggesting that the hippocampus and the MTLC support different aspects of recognition memory [3, 5, 6]. In particular, the hippocampus and the parahippocampal cortex were assumed to support recollection, i.e. recognition of an item on the basis of the retrieval of specific contextual details of the previous learning experience, whereas the perirhinal cortex subserves familiarity, i.e. item recognition on the basis of a scalar memory strength but without retrieval of any specific detail about the study episode.

These models, however, are hard to reconcile with the notion of a highly integrated network connecting all MTLC structures with each other and, most importantly, with the hippocampus [7]. Thus, more recent modifications sought to overcome the explanatory limitations of models associating MTLC and hippocampal functions in terms of the purely cognitive dichotomy between familiarity and recollection, respectively, by focusing on the kind of information, i.e. item-specific and contextual information, stored by the different substructures of the MTL [3, 8, 9]. Other models emphasize the putative operational characteristics of specific brain regions to describe the role of these regions in memory [7, 10]. The present chapter reviews evidence from animal research, neuropsychological studies with patients suffering from amnesia, and the growing body of neuroimaging studies that form the basis of each of the different accounts of the role of the hippocampus in memory.

Cognitive Processes Accounts

Following a widely acknowledged cognitive view, it has been argued that the hippocampus is vital for recognition based on recollection, but not for recognition based on familiarity (fig. 1a). These models usually further argue that MTLC regions (especially the perirhinal cortex, but not the parahippocampal cortex) are essential for familiarity-based recognition, and that this function is independent of the hippocampus [3, 11]. Consistent with this view, patients with severe hypoxic damage to the hippocampus exhibit disproportional large deficits in associative recognition (thought to rely on recollection) as compared to simple item memory (relying on familiarity, e.g. [12]). An almost identical pattern of impaired recollection and preserved familiarity has also been observed in a patient with selective hippocampal atrophy caused by meningitis [13]. The most striking evidence in favor of dual-process models comes from a double dissociation between deficits in recollection or associative memory following hippocampal damage compared to deficits in familiarity or item memory following damage to the perirhinal cortex [14]. These observations are paralleled by several animal stud-

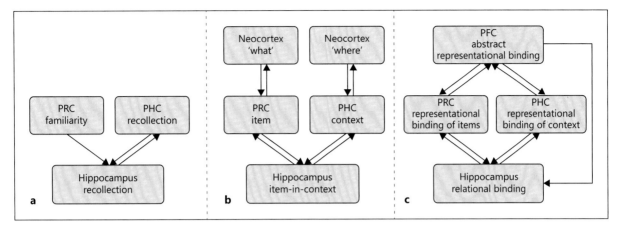

Fig. 1. Schematic illustrations of the core assumptions of cognitive processes accounts (**a**), informa-tion-based accounts (**b**), and neural processes-based accounts (**c**) (compare the role of different sub-structures within the MTL in memory). PRC = Perirhinal cortex; PHC = parahippocampal cortex; PFC = prefrontal cortex.

ies demonstrating that rats, initially trained to recognize associations between an odor (e.g. cumin, lemon, and thyme) and one of several digging media (e.g. sand, wood chips, etc.) and then retested after selective damage to the hippocampus, exhibited impaired recollection of the associations while memory for the odors alone was spared indicating intact familiarity [15]. In the same vein, neuroimaging studies in healthy participants employing associative recognition memory task demonstrated greater hippocampal activity for successful as compared to failed source recollection [16]. In this experiment, participants studied a word list while alternating between a pleasant/ unpleasant decision and a concrete/abstract decision. At test, they were required to discriminate between two simultaneously presented test words by selecting the mem-ber of the pair previously associated with a particular encoding task. Successful source retrieval was associated with increased activity in the left hippocampus.

Another method capitalizes on receiver operating characteristics, assuming that recollection is a threshold process whereas familiarity varies in a continuous manner with response confidence [17]. Therefore, a number of studies have used linear and curvi-linear approximations of confidence ratings (representing recollection and fa-miliarity, respectively) to identify regions where hemodynamic activity systematically varies with recognition confidence [18–20]. Such parametric analyses have consistent-ly shown that hippocampal activity is related to recollection. While some studies have found increasing activity in the perirhinal cortex as perceived strength of familiarity increased [18], others have reported monotonic decreases in activity with increasing memory strength not only in the perirhinal cortex, but also in the anterior hippocam-pus [19]. Yet another result was reported in a recent study [20] observing both decreas-ing and increasing activity as a function of increasing familiarity in the anterior and posterior perirhinal cortex, respectively. This latter finding emphasizes the contradictory results with respect to the role the MTLC plays in recognition memory.

A prominent alternative view explains the functional distinction between the hippocampus and adjacent MTLC structures described above with a single cognitive process in which differences in memory strength account for the differential involvement of the hippocampus and the perirhinal and parahippocampal cortices [2, 4]. While a weak memory trace seems sufficient to engage the MTLC, strong memories are required to engage the more powerful computational properties of the hippocampus. Evidence for this view is, for example, provided by studies demonstrating that amnesic patients are similarly impaired in all kinds of declarative memory [21]. However, single process models cannot account for the double dissociations in amnesia and neuroimaging studies cited above, nor can single process theories account for the double dissociations between the role of the hippocampus and the surrounding MTLC in recollection and familiarity in recent animal studies.

Information-Based Accounts

More recent models move beyond the simple and rather phenomenological dichotomy between recollection and familiarity towards an understanding of MTL functions in terms of the information they store. As depicted in figure 1b, these models propose that the perirhinal and the parahippocampal cortex support the encoding and retrieval of item-specific and contextual information, respectively, whereas the hippocampus stores representations of item-context associations [3, 8, 9]. This view is based on increased hippocampal activity in tasks emphasizing conjunctive memory representations such as memorizing paired associates [22], source memory tasks [23], and tasks requiring the spatial location of a previously presented item to be remembered [24]. In many of those studies, conversely, activity in the perirhinal cortex correlates with item rather than conjunctive memory performance [22, 24]. Together, these studies demonstrated that an increase of activity of the hippocampus is essential for the process of relating an item to contextual information during retrieval. This notion has gained further support from neuropsychological studies in amnesic patients [25, 26]. For instance, it was demonstrated that amnesic patients could discriminate between old and new visual scenes, but were unable to distinguish between intact old scenes and manipulated old scenes (e.g. by left-right shifting of particular elements within the scene) [26], indicating a deficit in processing the relations of items within a specific context rather than a deficit in recollection, per se.

Parallel evidence has also been obtained from animal studies showing that hippocampal neurons develop representations of the specific combination of stimulus elements (odors A and B) and the context (rooms X and Y) in which they occur [27]. In the beginning of their training, the rats' hippocampal neurons responded selectively to a specific location in the environment occupied by the animals (so-called 'place cells'). However, after several exposures to the same contextual discrimination problem, i.e. odor A is only rewarded in room X, when the animals acquired the item-context associations, some neurons began to fire selectively during the sampling of a specific item in a particular context and these cells continued to exhibit item-context specificity after learning. Similar firing patterns for the combination of specific stimuli with a location or behavioral context in which they occurred has also been demonstrated for monkeys [28] and humans [29]. These results indicate that hippocampal firing patterns reflect unique conjunctions of stimuli with the places and contexts in which the stimuli occur. Extending this view, it has also been proposed that associations of multiple items that share their cortical representations due to a substantial feature overlap (within the same domain, e.g. two faces or two words) can be stored by the perirhinal cortex and recognized based on their familiarity [30]. Evidence for this assumption comes from several neuropsychological patients with selective hippocampal damage who demonstrated severe impairments in the recognition of, for example, object-location and face-voice associations, while they were relatively unimpaired at recognizing pairs of words, nonwords, and unknown and famous faces after one or several study trials [31].

Common to all the examples described above and more general to typical episodic memory tasks, the item presented at the time of learning has to be associated with its specific study context. Later during recognition this association must be retrieved. As argued above, the hippocampus enables the retrieval of the association of an item with its study context and, consequently, will lead to the phenomenological experience of recollection. In contrast, the proposed role of the perirhinal cortex in retrieving item information alone is in agreement with the dual-process view of familiarity-based recognition. Thus, recollection and familiarity can be regarded as rather epiphenomenal to the information processed within the hippocampus and the MTLC, respectively.

Neural Process-Based Accounts

In a similar vein, others have proposed that functional differences between MTL sub-regions are based on their key computational role in memory [7, 10, 32]. Despite their differences, these views about MTL functions converge on the opinion that the distinct properties of hippocampal neurons and neurons in the surrounding MTLC subserve different memory processes (fig. 1c). It was suggested that sparse neural coding within the hippocampus will (1) foster the convergence of disparate cortical representations of items, actions, etc., and their spatiotemporal context that compose a unique input into a bound representation of that input and will (2) reduce the probability that the same neurons within the hippocampus are activated by two different inputs, thereby leading to distinct (pattern-separated) representations [10, 32]. The process of binding mentioned in (1) can be specified in terms of relational operations (e.g. identity, greater than or earlier than) that link together and organize the individual elements of an experience. For example, during paired associate learning, two items provide relational information about their identity with respect to their spatio-temporal context that is processed by the hippocampus. The hippocampus is capable to organize any arbitrary relation, which is a very effortful but highly flexible process. Consequently, it allows for the rearrangement of the elements of individual experiences to deal with novel situations. Crucially, the hippocampal circuitry possesses anatomical and computational characteristics to support these properties of separated relational bindings (see [3], for a detailed discussion). Due to this separation of different inputs mentioned in (2) the hippocampus is able to entirely reconstruct each single input (pattern completion), e.g. an item bound to its study context. It thereby enables the retrieval of contextual information. Thus, the process of relational binding will lead to recognition based on recollection. This close connection between relational binding and recollection was corroborated by animal studies and neuroimaging studies (extensively reviewed by [3, 9]).

In contrast, the neural activity of separate inputs to the MTLC is highly overlapping and therefore allows processing the shared structure of these separate inputs (representational bindings). For example, the first presentation of an item in a particular context, e.g. during encoding, weakly activates a large number of MTLC neurons, whereas repeated and thus familiar stimuli, although in a different context (e.g. during a recognition test), activate only a subset of these neurons representing the familiar stimuli, but with every neuron activated to a stronger degree [32]. Thus, during recognition, the presentation of a studied item initiates a set of processes that may be described in a more cognitive framework as a comparison between the neural activity associated with the short-lived representation of the actual stimulus and the confined activity in the MTLC of the previous encounter of that stimulus. As a result, a scalar familiarity signal is provided that tracks the global similarity between the test probe and the studied items [33]. It should be noted that similar to the information-based accounts it is assumed that, due to the divergent neural connections of the MTLC subregions to neocortical areas, different structures within the MTLC bind different features of the entire input [7, 34]. While the perirhinal cortex encodes information about objects, the parahippocampal cortex represents the respective context of that input (fig. 1c).

As a consequence of this representational binding, the MTLC is capable of extracting the general regularities inherent in the input over repeated exposures to that input. These regularities mainly comprise frequency of cooccurrence, but may also include transition probabilities or temporal contingencies (e.g. red and green in a traffic light, or item positions in a list-learning paradigm). However, there are limitations to the ability of the MTLC to abstract the regularities inherent in the recent input. As the MTLC receives the majority of its inputs from unimodal and polymodal association areas [34], representational bindings within the MTLC are necessarily based on superficial perceptual features. Consequently, the MTLC is hardly capable of creating abstract representations that are essential for goal-directed behavior. However, the prefrontal cortex seems ideally suited for the abstraction of such behavior-guiding representations [35]. Thus, while the MTLC mainly binds the representation of the actual item/context to the representation of a previous occurrence of that same item/ context, the prefrontal cortex mediates the binding of the actual event to a more abstract or prototypical representation of invariant and nonaccidental features of that event.

This binding view is supported by recent studies demonstrating an impairment of patients with anterior MTL lesions, including the perirhinal cortex, in perceptual discrimination of complex objects with a large number of overlapping features [36]. More importantly, this impairment was largest for objects with preexisting semantic representations, e.g. beasts as compared to novel objects such as bar codes. This is consistent with the present view that representational bindings supported by the perirhinal cortex link the actual appearance of a particular object to the mental representation of previous experiences with that same object. In a similar vein, the parahippocampal cortex mediates representational bindings of contextual features. For instance, it was demonstrated that the parahippocampal cortex is more active for objects that are strongly associated with a specific context (e.g. roulette wheel) than for objects that are very weakly associated with many possible contexts (e.g. cherry) [37]. These examples underscore the important role of both cortices for representational binding by demonstrating that readdressing object and/or contextual features of object occurrence during the repeated processing of a particular event require the integrity/activity of perirhinal and parahippocampal cortex, respectively.

Conclusion

The present chapter summarizes part of the recent evidence for the role of the hippocampus and the surrounding MTLC in memory. Several accounts have described hippocampal function in terms of the cognitive processes subserved by different substructures within the MTL, while others have focused more on the different information processed by these structures or on the underlying neural operations. Although accounts based on the dichotomy between recollection and familiarity have a long-standing tradition in memory research, it is still an open question whether the brain actually operates on this dichotomy. The two other accounts are more directly related to the different structures and the respective neural processes. While the exact relation of the neural processes to the assumed cognitive processes remains to be clarified, it seems that the neural processes account cuts across the boundaries inherent in the cognitive processes.

The list of accounts on hippocampal memory function is far from complete. Other accounts implicate the hippocampus in recent, but not in remote, memories. These are special cases of the overarching issue of memory consolidation, assuming that under certain circumstances memories can become independent of the hippocampus. Although these circumstances are subject to current debate, they are of high importance for amnesia research. Yet others emphasize the role of the hippocampus in spatial memory. More generally, these highly different views are suggestive of a more general role of MTL substructures in memory than discussed in the present chapter.

It should be also noted that the hippocampus and the perirhinal and parahippocampal cortices are interconnected with multiple brain areas in the parietal and frontal lobes. As the focus of this chapter was on the role of the hippocampus in memory, the important contribution of these other brain structures was not covered. However, only when their role is taken into account can a more complete picture of the importance of the MTL for the formation of declarative memories be drawn.

References

1 Scoville WB, Milner B: Loss of recent memory after bilateral hippocampal lesions. J Neurol Neurosurg Psychiatry 1957;20:11–21.
2 Wixted JT, Squire LR: The medial temporal lobe and the attributes of memory. Trends Cogn Sci 2011;15: 210–217.
3 Eichenbaum HB, Yonelinas AP, Ranganath C: The medial temporal lobe and recognition memory. Annu Rev Neurosci 2007;30:123–152.
4 Squire LR, Wixted JT, Clark RE: Recognition memory and the medial temporal lobe: a new perspective. Nat Rev Neurosci 2007;8:872–883.
5 Davachi L, Wagner AD: Hippocampal contributions to episodic encoding: insights from relational and item-based learning. J Neurophysiol 2002;88:982–990.
6 Diana RA, Yonelinas AP, Ranganath C: The effects of unitization on familiarity-based source memory: testing a behavioral prediction derived from neuroimaging data. J Exp Psychol Learn Mem Cogn 2008; 34:730–740.
7 Aggleton JP: Multiple anatomical systems embedded within the primate medial temporal lobe: implications for hippocampal function. Neurosci Biobehav Rev 2012;36:1579–1596.
8 Davachi L: Item, context and relational episodic encoding in humans. Curr Opin Neurobiol 2006;16: 693–700.
9 Diana RA, Yonelinas AP, Ranganath C: Imaging recollection and familiarity in the medial temporal lobe: a three-component model. Trends Cogn Sci 2007;11: 379–386.
10 Opitz B: Neural binding mechanisms in learning and memory. Neurosci Biobehav Rev 2010;34:1036–1046.
11 Brown MW, Aggleton JP: Recognition memory: what are the roles of the perirhinal cortex and hippocampus? Nat Rev Neurosci 2001;2:51–61.
12 Yonelinas AP, Quamme JR, Widaman KF, Kroll NEA, Sauvéand MJ, Knight RT: Mild hypoxia disrupts recollection, not familiarity. Cogn Affect Behav Neurosci 2004;4:393–400.
13 Aggleton JP, Vann SD, Denby C, Dix S, Mayes AR, Roberts N, Yonelinas AP: Sparing of the familiarity component of recognition memory in a patient with hippocampal pathology. Neuropsychologia 2005;43: 1810–1823.
14 Bowles B, Crupi C, Mirsattari SM, Pigott SE, Parrent AG, Pruessner JC, Yonelinas AP, Köhler S: Impaired familiarity with preserved recollection after anterior temporal-lobe resection that spares the hippocampus. Proc Natl Acad Sci USA 2007;104:16382–16387.
15 Fortin NJ, Wright SP, Eichenbaum H: Recollection-like memory retrieval in rats is dependent on the hippocampus. Nature 2004;431:188–191.
16 Dobbins IG, Rice HJ, Wagner AD, Schacter DL: Memory orientation and success: separable neurocognitive components underlying episodic recognition. Neuropsychologia 2003;41:318–333.
17 Yonelinas AP: The nature of recollection and familiarity: a review of 30 years of research. J Mem Lang 2002;46:441–517.
18 Montaldi D, Spencer TJ, Roberts N, Mayes AR: The neural system that mediates familiarity memory. Hippocampus 2006;16:504–520.
19 Daselaar SM, Fleck MS, Cabeza R: Triple dissociation in the medial temporal lobes: recollection, familiarity, and novelty. J Neurophysiol 2006;96:1902–1911.
20 Yassa MA, Stark CEL: Multiple signals of recognition memory in the medial temporal lobe. Hippocampus 2008;18:945–954.

21 Holdstock JS, Mayes AR, Roberts N, Cezayirli E, Isaac CL, O'Reilly RC: Under what conditions is recognition spared relative to recall after selective hippocampal damage in humans? Hippocampus 2002; 12:341–351.

22 Kirwan CB, Stark CEL: Medial temporal lobe activation during encoding and retrieval of novel face-name pairs. Hippocampus 2004;14:919–930.

23 Davachi L, Mitchell JP, Wagner AD: Multiple routes to memory: distinct medial temporal lobe processes build item and source memories. Proc Natl Acad Sci USA 2003;100:2157–2162.

24 Uncapher MR, Otten LJ, Rugg MD: Episodic encoding is more than the sum of its parts: an fMRI investigation of multifeatural contextual encoding. Neuron 2006;52:547–556.

25 Mayes AR, Holdstock JS, Isaac CL, Montaldi D, Grigor J, Gummer A, Cariga P, Downes JJ, Tsivilis D, Gaffan D, Gong Q, Norman KA: Associative recognition in a patient with selective hippocampal lesions and relatively normal item recognition. Hippocampus 2004;14:763–784.

26 Ryan JD, Althoff RR, Whitlow S, Cohen NJ: Amnesia is a deficit in relational memory. Psychol Sci 2000;11: 454–461.

27 Komorowski RW, Manns JR, Eichenbaum H: Robust conjunctive item-place coding by hippocampal neurons parallels learning what happens where. J Neurosci 2009;29:9918–9929.

28 Wirth S, Yanike M, Frank LM, Smith AC, Brown EN, Suzuki WA: Single neurons in the hippocampus and learning of new associations. Science 2003;300: 1578–1581.

29 Ekstrom AD, Kahana MJ, Caplan JB, Fields TA, Isham EA, Newman EL, Fried I: Cellular networks underlying human spatial navigation. Nature 2003;425: 184–187.

30 Mayes AR, Montaldi D, Migo E: Associative memory and the medial temporal lobes. Trends Cogn Sci 2007;11:126–135.

31 Mayes AR, Holdstock JS, Isaac CL, Hunkin NM, Roberts N: Relative sparing of item recognition memory in a patient with adult-onset damage limited to the hippocampus. Hippocampus 2002;12:325–340.

32 O'Reilly RC, Norman KA: Hippocampal and neocortical contributions to memory: advances in the complementary learning systems approach. Trends Cogn Sci 2002;6:505–510.

33 Hintzman DL: Similarity, global matching, and judgments of frequency. Mem Cognit 2001;29:547–556.

34 Suzuki WA, Amaral DG: Functional neuroanatomy of the medial temporal lobe memory system. Cortex 2004;40:220–222.

35 Simons JS, Spiers HJ: Prefrontal and medial temporal lobe interactions in long-term memory. Nat Rev Neurosci 2003;4:637–648.

36 Barense MD, Gaffan D, Graham KS: The human medial temporal lobe processes online representations of complex objects. Neuropsychologia 2007;45: 2963–2974.

37 Bar M, Aminoff E: Cortical analysis of visual context. Neuron 2003;38:258–347.

Prof. Dr. Bertram Opitz
School of Psychology, University of Surrey
Guildford GU2 7XH (UK)
E-Mail b.opitz@surrey.ac.uk

Szabo K, Hennerici MG (eds): The Hippocampus in Clinical Neuroscience.
Front Neurol Neurosci. Basel, Karger, 2014, vol 34, pp 60–70 (DOI: 10.1159/000356425)

Neuropsychological Measures of Hippocampal Function

Manon Wicking · Frauke Nees · Frauke Steiger

Department of Cognitive and Clinical Neuroscience, Central Institute of Mental Health, Medical Faculty Mannheim, Heidelberg University, Mannheim, Germany

Abstract

The role of the medial temporal lobe, specifically the hippocampus, in learning and memory has been consistently demonstrated over the past years and has led to the identification of the hippocampus as a target imaging marker for several neurological and psychiatric disorders. Hippocampal dysfunctions and smaller hippocampal volumes have been reported as characteristic for these disorders, and hippocampal asymmetry has been shown to be associated with memory deficits in older adults. These findings underline the importance of screenings for memory functions using neuropsychological cognitive test batteries within the clinical context. To the best of our knowledge, there has been no comprehensive review that has presented neuropsychological tests related to the hippocampus in detail. However, we did not aim to provide a complete overview of neuropsychological tests related to hippocampal function, which would fail in the light of the widespread area. This chapter focuses on neuropsychological tests that assess cognitive functions that depend on the hippocampus in a state-of-the-art fashion and additionally provide the link to several disorders for which hippocampal abnormalities are a common characteristic.

© 2014 S. Karger AG, Basel

The hippocampus plays an important role in learning, memory, and spatial navigation. The hippocampal formation has been implicated in a large number of disorders, from neurological disorders such as Alzheimer's disease, temporal lobe epilepsy, transient global amnesia, and cognitive ageing to mental disorders involving schizophrenia, depression, posttraumatic stress disorder, and other anxiety disorders. Over the years, three main neuropsychological theories of hippocampal function have been developed, related to inhibition, memory, and spatial function.

Neuropsychological assessment aims to assess the extent to which a particular skill is impaired and to determine the brain region that may have been damaged. Most neuropsychological tests not only assess one specific domain or skill component, but traditionally assess multiple skills and functions in several domains involving language, perception, intelligence, executive functions, and memory that can dissociate in the pathological brain. Likewise, hippocampal dysfunction does not result in one circumscribed deficit. The identification and quantification of deficits in cognitive functions derived from neuropsychological tests further allow the specification of dysfunctional processes that are characteristic for a certain disorder. From those tests, especially pertaining to the hippocampus, memory tests are used to assess functions related to processes of declarative memory, involving (context-dependent) episodic memory (i.e. the recollection of experiences and episodes), semantic memory (i.e. knowledge of the world), and procedural memory (i.e. remembering how to undertake tasks). Such neuropsychological testing situations involve learning, recognition, and recall of different material (e.g. related to allocentric spatial information and navigation).

Through decades of experience, standard neuropsychological tests have been developed which are sensitive to hippocampal function and are now used in nearly all studies investigating the effect of several disorders. For example, Alzheimer's disease or ischemic vascular dementia can reliably be dissociated using tests of procedural memory and declarative memory [1]. In addition, progressive and interrelated structural-functional hippocampal deficits have been demonstrated for schizophrenia. Here, cognitive deficits related to the hippocampus represent risk factors for an increase in psychotic symptoms. They can for example be assessed via tests of free recall and recognition performance [2]. These findings underline the importance of neuropsychological testing related to hippocampal function not only for a better understanding of hippocampus-dependent cognitive, learning, and memory processes, but more importantly within a clinical context. Although there are a few studies that have linked hippocampal function to executive and motor functioning, in the present chapter we focus on memory and visuospatial tests since the majority of studies are related to these functions.

Memory

It is well known that multiple memory systems exist in humans that distinguish between short-term or working memory and long-term memory. The latter is divided into the explicit (declarative: episodic and semantic) memory and the implicit (procedural or nondeclarative) memory. Damage to the hippocampus can result in anterograde amnesia (i.e. having difficulties forming new memories), as well as in retrograde amnesia to some extent, i.e. affecting memories that were formed years before the damage while very old memories largely remain [3].

The declarative memory system is the system that is most consistently shown to depend on hippocampal function. Recent research suggests that the hippocampal formation is involved in certain aspects of episodic memory. Episodic memory can be mainly subdivided in two processes, recollection and familiarity. When a subject recollects an event he or she consciously remembers the time, the context, and all the different elements about the episode. This leads to reliving of a previously experienced event. In contrast, familiarity refers to the kind of memory when one recognizes something without having this context information. For example, the face of a stranger can be familiar to you, but you cannot recollect when and where you have met that person for the first time. Eldridge et al. [4] for example showed hippocampal activity only when retrieval was accompanied by conscious recollection of the learning and not for items recognized based on familiarity. Similarly interesting is the question of whether – and to what extent – the hippocampus is involved in encoding versus retrieval processes. Neuroimaging studies have demonstrated that hippocampal activity reflects both encoding as well as recollection processes. More specifically, Eldridge et al. [5] found that regions early in the hippocampal circuits such as the dentate gyrus and CA fields 2 and 3 were active during episodic encoding and that the subiculum was more active during the recollection of the learning episode.

Memory tests are most frequently divided into verbal, visual, and behavioral memory functions. Among verbal memory, the most frequently used tests refer to story recall and list-learning. After reading a short local news story, the subjects are asked to recall as much details as possible after different time windows, e.g. immediately after they have read the story and again 30 min to an hour later. In list-learning tests, individuals have to learn a list of for example 15–20 words over a number of trials. For these words, they are then tested in recall and/or recognition sessions following distraction or delay. Behavioral tests consist of nonverbal material such as complex figures or designs. Here, an individual is required to reproduce as much as possible from a complex geometric figure that he or she has seen immediately or up to an hour before (see details below). Such behavioral memory tests have the advantage of being more ecologically valid because the test skills are needed in everyday life. To sum this up, semantic memory is assessed via category listing, verbal fluency tests, or picture naming, and episodic memory is assessed via asking an individual to recall or recognize previously learned information such as words, stories, or pictures.

When testing episodic memory performance, there is a need for easy applicable memory tests that have the ability to differentiate between the constructs described above. As mentioned above, most commonly used measures of episodic memory rely on recollection processes and include free recall, cued recall, and recognition of lists of items. In the following paragraphs, the most common neuropsychological tests of episodic memory are described.

Memory-based tests of symptom validity are designed to assess cognitive ability and are sensitive to performance in patients with severe neurological diseases that might show strong impairments which makes an interpretation along recommended cutoff scores more challenging. In the Word Memory Test [e.g., 6], individuals have to learn a list of 20 semantically linked pairs of common words, with its recognition, paired associate, multiple-choice, consistency, and free-recall subtest components. This test is one example that is designed to assess verbal declarative memory processes and thus processes related to the medial temporal lobe, specifically the hippocampus [6]. It is therefore also particularly sensitive for assessing memory performance in individuals with hippocampal damage such as amnestic patients.

The most sophisticated and widely used verbal episodic memory test is the California Verbal Learning Test-II (CVLT-II) [7]. The CVLT-II assesses explicit recall and recognition of semantically related words presented over multiple trials. It is especially useful because it analyzes different components of learning and memory which is important to characterize memory profiles in different mental disorders. This test assesses overall achievement and qualitative aspects of performance, such as learning strategies and error types. Recent research has shown that gender and left hippocampal volume are among the main predictors for verbal memory function in normal aging, the CVLT-Long Delay score was shown to correlate with hippocampal volume [8]. Impaired declarative memory performance and smaller hippocampal volume have also been observed in young and middle-aged adults with chronic posttraumatic stress disorder.

Similarly to the CVLT-II, the Wechsler Memory Scale-III [9] is one of the most popular memory tests among neuropsychologists. It assesses auditory and visual working and declarative memory and includes eleven subtests, six of which are considered as primary tests and the rest as optional. The test is sensitive for detecting verbal memory deficits in developmental disorders, like attention deficit hyperactivity disorder as well as memory deficits in Alzheimer's disease, Parkinson's disease, and Huntington's disease. For example, in a study of Brück et al. [10], the performance of patients with Parkinson's disease who showed left hippocampus atrophy correlated with verbal memory impairments.

In comparison, the Hopkins Verbal Learning Test (HVLT-R) [11] assesses verbal learning and memory in a brief fashion and has been validated within brain-disordered populations (e.g. Alzheimer's disease, amnestic disorders). The advantage of the test is its shortness and therefore it is useful for patients who are difficult to test and/or severely impaired. It consists of three learning trials, a delayed recall trial, and a delayed recognition trial. In sum, the HVLT-R seems to be a recommendable tool to distinguish between demented/amnestic groups and normal elderly [12].

Another example of a psychological memory test is the Rey Auditory Verbal Learning Test (RAVLT) [13], which assesses auditory-verbal memory, specifically the rate of learning, learning strategies, retroactive and proactive interference, presence of confabulation or confusion in memory processes, and retrieval of information. Participants are given a list of 15 unrelated words repeated over five different trials and are asked to reproduce all the words. Another list of 15 unrelated words is given and the client has to reproduce the original list immediately and after a 30-min delay. The RAVLT identified various patterns of deficits in different patient groups like amnestics or brain trauma injuries. There was a significant correlation between hippocampal volumes and scores on RAVLT in a study of Marchiani et al. [14], confirming that medial temporal structures are closely associated with memory performance in normal ageing as well as in amnestic mild cognitive impairment and Alzheimer's disease.

The Rivermead Behavioural Memory Test II (RBMT-II) [15] is yet another memory tool that sets itself apart from the other measurements through its real-life tasks. It is designed to mimic everyday duties that patients encounter to independently manage their lives. Compared to the conventional tasks of the RBMT-II, the real-life tasks show a greater correlation with psychosocial competence in patients which is necessary to assess in clinical settings. The RBMT-II is able to assess everyday memory function and can also be used as a monitoring tool to detect change over time. It was initially designed for the assessment of memory recovery in brain-injured patients. Low scores in the RBMT have been shown in patients with a variety of different disorders, e.g. dementia, alcohol-related disorders, and schizophrenia. It has been shown that it is not suitable for detecting mild or moderate memory impairments but can detect moderate-to-severe impairments [16].

To assess both verbal and visual memory components, the Recognition Memory Test (RMT) [17] is recommended. It contains tasks of recognition memory for printed words and photographs of faces. The RMT seems to be useful for detecting dementia especially in patients under 80 years of age, but is not sensitive enough for mild memory deficits. In a study by Bird and Burgess [18], two subtests of the RMT allowed them to investigate whether or not recognition-memory deficits are a pervasive feature of hippocampal amnesia or whether performance depends upon the nature of the task material. The recognition memory of patients with a bilateral damage to the hippocampus is impaired for words but intact for faces. The explanation of the authors suggests that the hippocampus boosts recognition of well-known stimuli (high-frequency words) by activating preexperimental associations that enrich the context of their presentation. In contrast, recognition memory for some kinds of previously unfamiliar stimuli (unfamiliar faces) may be supported by extrahippocampal familiarity-based processes.

Interestingly, some studies investigated the direct relationship of hippocampal volume and neuropsychological tests for memory performance involving the Wechsler Memory Scale, the National Adult Reading Test, the Wisconsin Card Sorting Test, or the Mini-Mental State Examination, a neuropsychological tool that has been shown to be associated with hippocampal volume, specifically the right hippocampal volume. The latter test assesses major domains of cognitive functioning involving memory, language, and visuospatial ability, and is used to differentiate amnestic mild cognitive impairment from normal ageing. Although some studies did not find significant associations, other studies, for example using samples of schizophrenia patients, showed positive association of logical memory with left anterior hippocampal volumes but of declarative episodic memory with reduced hippocampal volume [19]. Such inconsistencies across studies could be related on the one hand to whole brain volume since some effects were dramatically reduced when whole brain volume was partialled out, but on the other hand could also be related to methodological differences or diagnostic issues.

Visuospatial Function

Spatial information processing depends on information from multiple brain areas in the parietal, temporal (including the hippocampus), and occipital lobes, mainly in the right hemisphere. Two main streams are supposed to represent visuospatial ability: an occipitotemporal stream (ventral system) responsible for object identification and an occipitoparietal stream (dorsal system) responsible for the spatial relationship between objects. Common neuropsychological tests for visuospatial function are 'block design' [9] and 'clock drawing' [20].

Block design is a subtest of one of the major neuropsychological test batteries, the Wechsler Memory Scale-III [9], that measures visuoconstructive abilities. The individual has to reproduce a spatial pattern that is presented on a card using three-dimensional two-colored blocks with different patterns. A similar test from the same battery is 'block tapping' that measures visuospatial memory span. It is a simple but powerful tool to examine a person's immediate spatial working memory. The apparatus usually consists of nine blocks arranged irregularly on a board. The examiner taps the blocks in a randomized sequence and the subject tries to reproduce that sequence immediately afterwards. This procedure is repeated with successively increasing length until the subject is no longer accurate.

Brain activity in healthy individuals during block tapping has recently been examined by Toepper et al. [21]. They presented their subjects with a modified version of the block tapping test in a functional magnetic resonance imaging (MRI) scanner. Hippocampal structures, especially the right hippocampus, were more activated during the block tapping condition and therefore seem to contribute to serial working memory encoding of spatial locations in the human brain. Patients with potential damage to the hippocampus, such as schizophrenia, show deficits in the storage and subsequent reproduction of spatial target sequences, which are the core functions for successful task performance. For example, it has been shown that schizophrenic patients and their unaffected co-twins perform significantly worse than control subjects on a block tapping task [22].

The impact of the hippocampus for visuoconstruction is also evident in clock drawing, a test that is used as a screening for cognitive impairment and as a measure of spatial dysfunction and neglect. Instructions for the test are simple: patients are asked to draw a clock, put in all the numbers and set the hands at ten past eleven. It has been shown that abnormal clock drawing occurs in neurodegenerative disorders such as vascular dementia and Alzheimer's disease. A recent study investigating subcortical morphological correlates of clock drawing performance showed that even though the volume and shape of several brain regions (amygdala, caudate nucleus, hippocampus, nucleus accumbens, pallidum, putamen, and thalamus) are related to task performance, impairments in clock drawing are predominantly associated with alterations in the bilateral hippocampus and in the right globus pallidus [23].

Another test that measures visuoconstructive skills and visual memory is the Rey-Osterrieth Complex Figure Test (RCFT) [24]. Here, subjects are required to reproduce an abstract line drawing in three steps: copy, immediate recall, and 30-min delayed recall. In a study investigating patients that underwent brain surgery in order to alleviate pharmacologically intractable epilepsy, right hippocampal damage was shown to be involved in immediate and delayed recall, but not in correct copying of the figure [25]. More recent studies, however, contradict those early findings. McConley et al. [24], for example, examined the association between figural and spatial components of the RCFT, temporal lobe laterality, and hippocampal structure using MRI hippocampal volumes and neuropathology ratings, but did not find an association between the hippocampus and immediate or delayed recall scores. This indicates that RCFT recall is a poor marker of right temporal lobe function in temporal lobectomy candidates.

The Benton Visual Retention Test (BVRT) [26] on the other hand has consistently been shown to directly measure hippocampal function. It is a widely used test for the evaluation of visuospatial memory, specifically visuoperception and visuoconstruction abilities. Subjects are presented with three sets of cards containing ten different geometric figures. The BVRT can be administered as a reproduction task, where the subject has to either copy the design while looking at the card or reproduce the design from memory immediately after presentation or after a 15-second delay ('administration format'). Furthermore, a 'multiple choice/recognition format' can be used. Here, participants view a visual pattern for 10 s and then have to identify the target stimulus from an array of four patterns. In a high-resolution variant of functional MRI, Brickman et al. [27] found that performance on the recognition component of the BVRT was associated with cerebral blood volume in the dentate gyrus – a part of the hippocampal formation. The study also showed that the elevation in blood glucose, a process that is known to target the dentate gyrus, correlates selectively with the recognition component of the BVRT. Hence, object recognition memory as part of the BVRT may represent a direct measure of hippocampal, and specifically dentate gyrus, function (fig. 1).

In addition to visuoconstruction abilities, object location learning (remembering the location of specific objects) and positional memory (remembering the precise metric coordinates without any item information) have also been shown to rely on the hippocampus. In a meta-analysis [28], patients with lesions of the hippocampal for-

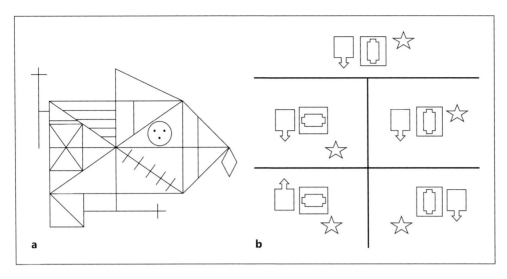

Fig. 1. a Rey-Osterrieth Complex Figure Test: Patients are asked to copy the figure, and asked to re-draw the figure from memory 30 min later. **b** Modified image from the Benton Visual Retention Test: the design at the top is presented and after a delay patients are asked to choose the one that best matches the original.

mation were impaired on four different types of spatial-memory tasks, including object location learning and positional memory. Object-location memory also revealed a lateralization of function: patients with lesions of the right hippocampus performed worse than patients with left hippocampal damage. There are several neuropsychological tests that measure visuospatial learning, such as object location and positional memory. In the Location Learning Test (LLT, e.g. [29]), patients are required to learn the correct placement of for example 10 everyday objects on a 5 x 5 grid, presented to them on a stimulus card, and can be tested in an immediate and a 30-min delayed recall condition. The LLT is presented in this chapter because it is a brief paper-pencil test that does not require fine motor control, verbal responses, or complex instructions and is therefore applicable to a wide range of patients, such as older adults, patients with dementia, and brain-damaged patients.

Most of the aforementioned tests primarily assess one specific visuospatial function. The Cambridge Neuropsychological Test Automated Battery (CANTAB; Cambridge Cognition) combines several tests that measure different spatial functions – among a variety of other cognitive skills – such as memory, attention, and executive function. Specifically, this nonverbal test battery offers tests of spatial memory and spatial orientation. Stimuli are abstract designs, delivered on a touch screen computer, tasks include recognizing a series of 24 patterns ('pattern recognition memory'), recognizing the position of a series of 20 squares ('spatial recognition memory'), and searching a number of boxes on a screen for hidden tokens ('spatial working memory'). It has been shown that older depressed subjects have persistent cognitive impairments as measured by various CANTAB tests (i.e. 'spatial span' and 'spatial working memory') that are associated with hippocampal volume reduction [30].

In addition to those rather explicit spatial abilities, the hippocampus has been shown to also be involved in implicit motor sequence learning. The Serial Reaction Time Task (SRTT), for example, is a popular method in neuropsychological research, and even though its use for clinical testing is limited, we believe that it should be mentioned, as it has been shown to reliably measure hippocampal function. In the SRTT, participants are asked to repeatedly respond to visual cues that can appear in one of four (or more) positions on a computer screen. Each screen position indicates that a particular response is to be made, i.e. a button press. What the participant does not know is that there is an underlying fixed sequence of positions on the screen and therefore of required button presses (i.e. 4-2-3-1-4-1-2-3-1-2-4-3) in some of the trials. With time, reaction times become increasingly shorter in the sequential trials, but not in the random trials. Research showed that the hippocampus and adjacent structures are involved in explicit and implicit learning of sequences. A recent study using single-trial intracranial EEG in presurgical epileptic patients identified the hippocampus as providing a major contribution to the reliable classification of the trained sequence with an additional contribution of frontostriatal regions [28].

Conclusion

In this chapter, we presented neuropsychological tests related to hippocampal function in a state-of-the-art fashion and additionally provided the link to disorders with hippocampal abnormalities as a common characteristic. The hippocampus plays a crucial role in memory and spatial navigation processes, and corresponding tests are of crucial importance when hippocampal function is to be addressed in neuropsychological assessment (i.e., for diagnostic purposes in disorders known to involve hippocampal damage). A mass of literature on different neuropsychological tests assessing memory and spatial functions exists, but to the best of our knowledge there is no consolidated report on neuropsychological tests specifically related to hippocampal function and its clinical application. This is not surprising because providing a comprehensive overview is highly challenging – not only would it underestimate the whole range of tests, but it would also lack specificity, as detailed examinations on the sensitivity of neuropsychological tests as clinical diagnostic tools with specific relation to the hippocampus are still missing. However, it is remarkable that research has enabled us to differentiate between different memory processes, such as encoding and retrieval, with rather simple neuropsychological tests. We do not only know that the hippocampus per se is involved, but also have an idea of the hippocampal substructures that underlie these processes.

With respect to the clinical field, it should be noted that studies identifying memory deficits as being very robustly associated to hippocampal lesions mainly investigated healthy individuals after focal lesions or patients with temporal lobe epilepsy. However, in disorders such as schizophrenia, abnormalities within the hippocampus might be the result of neurodevelopmental abnormalities rather than of acquired (focal) lesions, and neuropsychological deficits have to be interpreted more carefully, or at least within a different context.

Outlook

In the past, neuropsychological and neuroimaging studies have generally addressed the hippocampus as a single structure, but more recent studies have shown a rather complex pattern highlighting the importance of subregions for distinct cognitive operations in general as well as clinically relevant dysfunctions. For example, Brickman et al. [27] identified memory tests that are specifically associated with the dentate gyrus (BVRT) and the entorhinal cortex (Selective Reminding Test). From a neuropsychological perspective, the differential roles of hippocampal substructures become increasingly important in order to disentangle hippocampus-related (cognitive) dysfunctions not only in healthy individuals but more interestingly in patients suffering from different neurological and psychological disorders. The need to develop more sensitive neuropsychological tests seems warranted as they could serve as valuable diagnostic tools. A promising approach is the growing use of virtual reality technology in neuropsychological testing. Its various application possibilities offer new opportunities for the development of innovative assessment methods. As an example, tasks aiming at hippocampal (dys)function, such as tests of navigational skills, the ability to form and use cognitive maps of the environment, allocentric spatial memory, and context-dependent episodic memory, can take place in virtual towns or landscapes. Nevertheless, studies on the specific aspects of neuropsychological tests with respect to hippocampal function are still needed to further disentangle and comprise involved processes and structures.

References

1 Libon DJ, Bogdanoff B, Cloud BS, Skalina S, Giovannetti T, Gitlin HL, Bonavita J: Declarative and procedural learning, quantitative measures of the hippocampus, and subcortical white alterations in Alzheimer's disease and ischaemic vascular dementia. J Clin Exp Neuropsychol 1998;20: 30–41.

2 Helmstaedter C, Hoppe C, Elger CE: Memory alterations during acute high-intensity vagus nerve stimulation. Epilepsy Res 2001;47:37–42.

3 Squire LR, Schacter DL: The Neuropsychology of Memory. New York City, Guilford Press, 2002.

4 Eldridge LL, Engel SA, Zeineh MM, Bookheimer SY, Knowlton BJ: A dissociation of encoding and retrieval processes in the human hippocampus. J Neurosci 2005;25:3280–3286.

5 Eldridge LL, Knowlton BJ, Furmanski CS, Bookheimer SY, Engel SA: Remembering episodes: a selective role for the hippocampus during retrieval. Nat Neurosci 2000;3:1149–1152.

6 Ofen N, Kao YC, Sokol-Hessner P, Kim H, Whitfield-Gabrieli S, Gabrieli JD: Development of the declarative memory system in the human brain. Nat Neurosci 2007;10:1198–1205.

7 Delis DC, Kramer JH, Kaplan E, Ober BA: California Verbal Learning Test, ed 2, Adult Version. San Antonio, The Psychological Corporation, 2000.

8 Ystad MA, Lundervold AJ, Wehling E, Espeseth T, Rootwelt H, Westlye LT, Andersson M, Adolfsdottir S, Geitung JT, Fjell AM, Reinvang I, Lundervold A: Hippocampal volumes are important predictors for memory function in elderly women. BMC Med Imaging 2009;9:1–15.

9 Wechsler D: WMS-III Administration and Scoring Manual. San Antonio, The Psychological Corporation, 1997.

10 Brück A, Kurki T, Kaasinen V, Vahlberg T, Rinne JO: Hippocampal and prefrontal atrophy in patients with early non-demented Parkinson's disease is related to cognitive impairment. J Neurol Neurosurg Psychiatry 2004;75:1467–1469.

11 Brandt J, Benedict RHB: Hopkins Learning Verbal Test – Revised. Odessa, PAR, 2001.

12 Hogervorst E, Combrinck M, Lapuerta P, Rue J, Swales K, Budge M: The Hopkins Verbal Learning Test and screening for dementia. Dement Geriatr Cogn Disord 2002;13:13–20.

13 Schmidt M: Rey Auditory Verbal Learning Test. Los Angeles, Western Psychological Services, 1996.

14 Marchiani NCP, Balthazar MLF, Cendes F, Damasceno BP: Hippocampal atrophy and verbal episodic memory performance in amnestic mild cognitive impairment and mild Alzheimer's disease. A preliminary study. Dement Neuropsychol 2008;2:37–41.

15 Wilson BA, Cockburn J, Baddeley AD: The Rivermead Behavioural Memory Test. Bury St Edmunds, Thames Valley Test Company, 1985.

16 Strauss E, Sherman EMS, Spreen O: A Compendium of Neuropsychological Tests. New York, Oxford University Press, 2006.

17 Warrington EK: Recognition Memory Test Manual. Windsor, NFER-Nelson, 1984.

18 Bird CM, Burgess N: The hippocampus supports recognition memory for familiar words but not unfamiliar faces. Curr Biol 2008;18:1932–1936.

19 Nestor PG, Kubicki M, Kuroki N, Gurrera RJ, Niznikiewicz M, Shenton ME, McCarley RW: Episodic memory and neuroimaging of hippocampus and fornix in chronic schizophrenia. Psychiatry Res 2007;155:21–28.

20 Sunderland T, Hill JL, Mellow AM, Lawlor BA, Gundersheimer J, Newhouse PA, Grafman JH: Clock drawing in Alzheimer's disease. A novel measure of dementia severity. J Am Geriatr Soc 1989;37:725–729.

21 Toepper M, Markowitsch HJ, Gebhardt H, Beblo T, Thomas C, Gallhofer B, Driessen M, Sammer G: Hippocampal involvement in working memory encoding of changing locations: an fMRI study. Brain Res 2010;1354:91–99.

22 Pirkola T, Tuulio-Henriksson A, Glahn D, Kieseppä T, Haukka J, Kaprio J, Lönnqvist J, Cannon TD: Spatial working memory function in twins with schizophrenia and bipolar disorder. Biol Psychiatry 2005;58:930–936.

23 Seidl U, Traeger TV, Hirjak D, Remmele B, Wolf RC, Kaiser E, Stieltjes B, Essig M, Schröder J, Thomann PA: Subcortical morphological correlates of impaired clock drawing performance. Neurosci Lett 2012;512:28–32.

24 McConley R, Martin R, Palmer CA, Kuzniecky R, Knowlton R, Faught E: Rey Osterrieth complex figure test spatial and figural scoring: relations to seizure focus and hippocampal pathology in patients with temporal lobe epilepsy. Epilepsy Behav 2008;13:174–177.

25 Bohbot VD, Kalina M, Stepankova K, Spackova N, Petrides M, Nadel L: Spatial memory deficits in patients with lesions to the right hippocampus and to the right parahippocampal cortex. Neuropsychologia 1998;36:1217–1238.

26 Benton AL: A visual retention test for clinical use. Arch Neurol Psychiatry 1955;54:212–216.

27 Brickman AM, Stern Y, Small SA: Hippocampal subregions differentially associate with standardized memory tests. Hippocampus 2011;21:923–928.

28 De Lucia M, Constantinescu I, Sterpenich V, Pourtois G, Seeck M, Schwartz S: Decoding sequence learning from single-trial intracranial EEG in humans. PLoS One 2011;6:e28630.

29 Kessels RP, de Haan EH, Kappelle LJ, Postma A: Varieties of human spatial memory: a meta-analysis on the effects of hippocampal lesions. Brain Res Rev 2001;35:295–303.

30 O'Brien JT, Lloyd A, McKeith I, Gholkar A, Ferrier N: A longitudinal study of hippocampal volume, cortisol levels, and cognition in older depressed subjects. Am J Psychiatry 2004;161:2081–2090.

Frauke Nees, PhD
Department of Cognitive and Clinical Neuroscience
Central Institute of Mental Health, Square J 5
DE-68159 Mannheim (Germany)
E-Mail frauke.nees@zi-mannheim.de

Szabo K, Hennerici MG (eds): The Hippocampus in Clinical Neuroscience.
Front Neurol Neurosci. Basel, Karger, 2014, vol 34, pp 71–84 (DOI: 10.1159/000357925)

Conventional and Diffusion-Weighted MRI of the Hippocampus

Kristina Szabo[a] · Alex Förster[b] · Achim Gass[a]

Departments of [a]Neurology and [b]Neuroradiology, UniversitätsMedizin Mannheim, University of Heidelberg, Mannheim, Germany

Abstract

The human hippocampus is a highly complex structure located on the medial surface of the cerebral hemispheres as a part of the intralimbic gyrus. For clinical purposes, in addition to routine transverse MRI slices, acquisitions parallel and perpendicular to the long axis of the hippocampus need to be performed to fully appreciate its curved anatomy. Clinicians should be acquainted with the normal appearance of the hippocampus regarding size, shape, symmetry, and signal as well as with the width and form of the cerebrospinal fluid spaces surrounding the hippocampus to be able to recognize abnormalities. The human hippocampus can be affected in a variety of very different acute or chronic neurological diseases, such as stroke and certain forms of encephalitis or epilepsy and dementia. Many of these pathologies are associated with distinct lesion patterns on conventional MRI. In hippocampal sclerosis, the typical imaging features – T2 hyperintensity, atrophy on T1-weighted images, and disturbed internal structures of the hippocampus – can be reliably diagnosed by visual analysis. Several visual rating scales exist for the evaluation of medial temporal lobe atrophy for the assessment of patients with cognitive disturbances; however, quantitative MRI-based volumetric analysis is increasingly being applied in research as well as clinical studies. In acute neurological disorders, diffusion-weighted imaging has the ability to demonstrate even minute and transient hyperintense hippocampal lesions. On the basis of distinct lesions patterns, diffusion-weighted MRI can provide additional diagnostic information that may facilitate and support a final diagnosis, especially in those cases in which clinical symptoms are inconclusive.

In everyday clinical routine, special emphasis on imaging findings of the hippocampus is relevant in several typical settings. Basically, the hippocampus can be affected by very different pathologies in acute and chronic neurological disorders either in isolation or more commonly as a part of more extensive (visible) structural changes. In this chapter we will focus on clinically relevant aspects of MRI findings of the hippocampus using conventional and diffusion-weighted MRI sequences in common

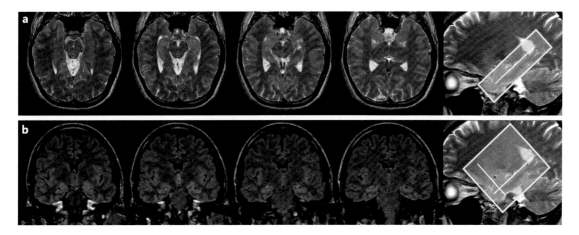

Fig. 1. MRI performed in two planes, parallel to the long axis of the hippocampus (T2-weighted example) (**a**) and perpendicular to the long axis of the hippocampus (FLAIR example) (**b**), enables the best anatomical assessment of this complex structure.

neurological disorders. Knowledge of the characteristic features of these – in many cases specific – hippocampal changes may give diagnostic clues and thus aid the clinician in differentiating the underlying pathology.

Anatomy of the Hippocampus on MRI

The hippocampus is part of the limbic lobe, more precisely of the intralimbic gyrus on the medial surface of the cerebral hemispheres (medial temporal lobe), and can be subdivided into three segments: the anterior head, the body, and the posterior tail. Due to its curved structure, the hippocampus is not readily appreciated on routine transverse MRI slices. MRI performed in two planes, (1) parallel to the long axis of the hippocampus and (2) in a slightly oblique coronal plane (perpendicular to the long axis of the hippocampus), enables the best anatomical assessment of this complex structure (fig. 1). A slice thickness of <3 mm with a 1-mm gap between slices is preferential. High resolution conventional or fast spin echo T2-weighted sequences and FLAIR images enable the evaluation of the internal architecture and signal changes, and additional diffusion-weighted images (DWI) should be performed in identical orientations. A 3-dimensional T1-weighted dataset (partition size ≤1.5 mm) allows for reformatting in any orientation, 3-dimensional reconstruction, and quantitative volumetry. For most of the entities discussed here, gadolinium enhancement is not of diagnostic value; however, it may be necessary if, for example, a neoplasm or an infection is suspected.

It is of course essential to be acquainted with the normal appearance of the hippocampus regarding size, shape, symmetry, and signal, as well as with the anatomy of the cerebrospinal fluid (CSF) spaces surrounding the hippocampus (perihippocampal fissures, uncal sulcus, and the hippocampal sulcus residual cavity), when evaluating MRIs for possible abnormalities. The perihippocampal fissures include the hippocampal fissure (or hippocampal sulcus, located between the dentate gyrus and the subiculum/CA1 field of the hippocampus), the lateral transverse fissure (lateral extension of the ambient cistern), the choroid fissure (superior lateral extension of the transverse fissure), and the temporal horn of the lateral ventricle [1]. The uncal sulcus is the part of the hippocampal fissure located ventral to the uncus. Hippocampal sulcus residual cavities (also termed hippocampal sulcal cavities) are remnants of the primitive hippocampal sulcus between the embryonic cornu ammonis and the dentate gyrus. Hippocampal sulcus residual cavities have been reported in over 50% of asymptomatic individuals; their prevalence is not believed to have a pathological value, whereas the sizes of the hippocampal fissure and the uncul sulcus correlate with age and atrophy [2, 3]. In an MRI study evaluating the hippocampus in healthy volunteers visually and qualitatively (as done in everyday clinical practice), the authors found that only mild variations occur with regard to hippocampal size and shape and hippocampal fissure visualization [4]. In more detail, they found no (80%) or only subtle (20%) subjective asymmetry of the hippocampus. In the coronal slice in the plane of the red nucleus, the shape of the hippocampal body was oval or rectangular, but never flattened. The hippocampal fissure and/or uncal sulcus was not larger than 1 mm in diameter. In addition, the normal hippocampal signal intensity is isointense to cortical gray matter on T1- and T2-weighted imaging and is slightly hyperintense to gray matter on FLAIR images.

Volumetric MRI Analysis of the Hippocampus

While qualitative (meaning visual) assessment is still the most commonly used approach to assess brain tissue loss and guide clinical decision-making in everyday routine, quantitative MRI-based volumetric analysis is increasingly being applied in research as well as in clinical studies to evaluate atrophy and morphometric changes of the brain, especially of the hippocampus. This development is the result of the fast and continuing advances in computational technologies and the development of automated software algorithms facilitating and accelerating the course of the analysis process. All in vivo volumetric techniques rely on image segmentation, i.e. partitioning an individual dataset into different structures of the brain, such as gray matter, white matter, CSF, or – as in this case – the hippocampus. As for the hippocampus, there is a wide range in the variety of protocols in use with differences in image acquisition, postacquisition processing, and volumetric analysis itself. These differences may in part explain some of the inconclusive and inconsistent results in hippocampal volumetric research findings [5].

Until recently, the manual outlining of the hippocampus along the anatomical boundaries according to empirical guidelines was considered the gold standard by

Table 1. Anatomical boundaries for manual segmentation of the hippocampus suggested by two commonly used protocols

	Cook et al. [42] (1992)	Jack [43] (1994)
Anterior border	alvear covering of hippocampal formation distinguishes amygdala from hippocampus	uncal recess or alveus
Posterior border	slice with greatest fornix length	crura of the fornices are fully seen
Medial border	open end of hippocampal and uncal fissures	CSF in the uncal and ambient cistern
Lateral border	not mentioned	CSF in the temporal horn
Inferior border	not mentioned	GM/WM junction between subiculum and WM in the PHG
Normative hippo-campal volume, cm^3		
Left	3.229	2.400
Right	3.185	2.800

GM = Gray matter; WM = white matter; PHG = parahippocampal gyrus.

many. Interestingly, even for this approach no standard protocol exists; instead there are approximately 60 varying guidelines that have been suggested and used by different groups [6, 7]. As examples for the variability in these guidelines, the anatomical boundaries reported in two frequently used protocols are shown in table 1. The disadvantages are obvious: this is a very time-consuming task that relies on a great amount of anatomical knowledge experience. In a collaborative effort, researchers from the European Alzheimer's Disease Consortium (EADC) and the Alzheimer's Neuroimaging Initiative (ADNI) are currently working on developing a harmonized manual segmentation protocol of the hippocampus [8].

In search of more objective measurements of the hippocampal volume, current methodologies employ semiautomated or fully automated techniques. This approach is more objective and of course especially advantageous when studying large patient populations; however, it might be hampered by interindividual anatomical differences, signal inhomogeneity, and partial volume effects [5].

MRI of the Hippocampus in Hippocampal Sclerosis

Hippocampal sclerosis (HS) is the most common pathologic finding in temporal lobe epilepsy patients undergoing surgery and was first described in histological postmortem studies as a finding associated with epilepsy under the name 'Ammon's horn scle-

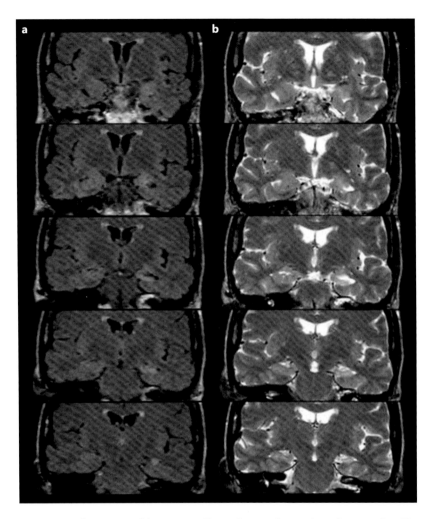

Fig. 2. MRI of a 61-year-old woman suffering from epilepsy since the age of 35. She reported having 2–5 partial and complex partial seizures per month. Coronal FLAIR (**a**, left column) and T2-weighted (**b**, right column) MRI shows atrophy and a hyperintense T2 signal of the left hippocampus as well as the amygdala consistent with HS.

rosis' by Sommer and Bratz in 1880 [9]. Since the early 1990s, it is acknowledged that MRI is able to detect HS [10]. The typical imaging features of HS – that can be reliably diagnosed by visual analysis – include increased T2-weighted signal, atrophy on T1-weighted images, and disturbed internal structures of the hippocampus (fig. 2). Increased signal on FLAIR images needs to be confirmed on T2-weighted images to rule out partial volume CSF effects. Atrophy and an increased T2 signal may be diffuse or regionally accentuated. Additional involvement of the neighboring temporal lobe structures, especially the amygdala and the parahippocampal gyrus may be present [11]. Internal disorganization is best appreciated on T1-weighted coronal inversion recovery images [12]. HS may be present in – mostly ipsilateral – extrahippocampal or extratemporal structural brain lesions, a finding termed 'dual pathology' [13]. It has been proposed that a primary vascular lesion, tumor, or cortical malformation may kindle HS.

MRI of the Hippocampus in Aging and Dementia

One of the most commonly faced questions in clinical neuroimaging practice is the evaluation of brain atrophy in elderly patients with mild cognitive impairment, different types of dementia, or other neuropsychiatric disorders. While historically used to exclude a cerebral lesion causing dementia, MRI is nowadays used to strengthen the clinical diagnosis. To measure brain atrophy, visual assessment, linear measurements, and volumetric calculation using a range of software tools can be applied. As quantitative measurements are generally too time consuming for routine clinical use, structured visual analysis scales have been proposed and should include visual assessment for the degree and pattern of global cortical atrophy, but also for focal atrophy in different brain regions including (among others) the medial temporal lobe. Scheltens et al. [14] have developed standard rating scales for all of these aspects. The visual rating scale for medial temporal lobe atrophy (published in 1992) is a score scale (0–4) to be used on coronal images T1-weighted images, and it assesses the maximal height of the hippocampal formation (hippocampus and parahippocampal gyrus) as well as the maximal width of the surrounding CSF spaces, namely the choroid fissure, and the temporal horn. Each one is rated as normal, increased, or decreased. However, since hippocampal volume declines even in healthy individuals as age increases, in older patients the normal range is larger than in younger ones. Several studies have shown good agreement with quantitative methods as well as good intrarater reliability of this fast and easy scale, and it has been shown that its use can distinguish early Alzheimer's disease patients from normal controls [14–16]. The scale was extended especially for application to patients with Alzheimer's disease and with frontotemporal dementia, taking into account the extrahippocampal temporal structures and validated by volumetric measures proposed by Galton et al. [17]. Other more specific rating scales include additional assessment of the entorhinal cortex and the inferior temporal gyrus or the frontal lobe. Table 2 describes disorders causing hippocampal atrophy, and figure 3 depicts an example of a patient with temporal atrophy in semantic dementia.

The advantages of MRI-based hippocampal volumetry for clinical use are multifold: the technique can be applied in clinical practice and research as a biomarker of neurological disease to support a diagnosis, to understand mechanism and track the clinical progression of disease, or to monitor treatment effects [5]. Most recently, the consistency of MRI measurements (obtained across sites and between multisite data) has suggested the technical feasibility of using structural MRI measures as a surrogate endpoint of disease progression in therapeutic trials [18]. It can be ex-

Table 2. Neurological disorders causing hippocampal atrophy

Etiology	Clinical features	Associated MRI findings
Alzheimer's disease	initial episodic memory loss; later: aphasia, apraxia; visuospatial deficits, executive dysfunction	posterior/parietal atrophy; bilateral, symmetrical; late hippocampal affection
Frontotemporal lobar degeneration/ frontotemporal dementia	aphasic and behavioral symptoms (according to subtype)	atrophy of temporal and frontal lobe; may be asymmetric
Dementia with Lewy bodies	scenic hallucinations; extrapyramidal symptoms	generalized cortical atrophy
HS	epilepsy	T2 hyperintensity; atrophy of amygdala and parahippocampal gyrus

pected that further refinement of high-field MRI data and new methods for image segmentation will increase the implementation of hippocampal volumetry into clinical routine.

Diffusion-Weighted Imaging of the Hippocampus

DWI was introduced and established as a routine imaging procedure in acute ischemic stroke in the late 1990s, and since then a large number of studies covering numerous different angles of ischemic stroke have been published. The lack of mobility of water protons as a consequence of cytotoxic edema in ischemic tissue lights up strongly against the dark background of healthy tissue on DWI, which provides a very high lesion-to-background contrast, and is seen as hypointensity on quantitative maps of the apparent diffusion coefficient (ADC). However, a hyperintense signal on DWI is not specific for brain tissue damage after acute ischemic stroke and, consequently, DWI studies in recent years have identified acute signal changes of brain tissue – and in particular of the hippocampus – in several other, quite different neurological disorders [19]. Knowledge of the characteristic features of these – in many cases specific – hippocampal changes may give diagnostic clues and thus aid the clinician in differentiating the underlying pathology (table 3).

Acute Ischemic Stroke

Acute ischemic stroke causes disruption of the cerebral energy metabolism, leading to failure of the Na^+/K^+ adenosine triphosphatase pump, a loss of ionic gradients and a net translocation of water from the extracellular to the intracellular compartments.

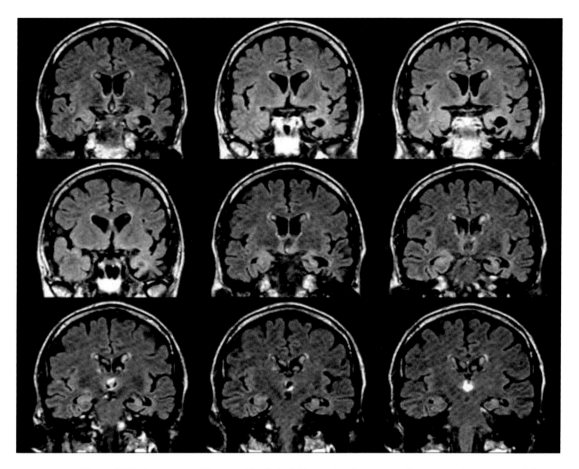

Fig. 3. MRI of a 64-year-old man with clinical diagnosis of semantic dementia who presented due to progressive word-finding difficulties since approximately 2 years. Neuropsychological evaluation revealed abnormalities of especially spontaneous speech and confrontational naming (including semantic and phonematic paraphasia, anomic aphasia) as well as comprehension difficulties and signs of executive dysfunction. Coronal FLAIR images show atrophy of the left hippocampus and the inferior anterior temporal lobe (fusiform gyrus and inferior temporal gyrus).

This is now the commonly accepted theory of restricted diffusion in acute stroke that leads to a high signal on DWI and a reduction of the ADC. Details of clinical and MRI findings in patients with acute ischemic stroke involving the hippocampus are given in Szabo [this vol., pp. 150–156].

Transient Global Amnesia

Transient global amnesia (TGA) is a neurological disorder characterized by a sudden onset of antero- and retrograde amnesia, and a complete recovery from this cognitive disturbance within 24 h (for an extensive overview of the disorder see Szabo [this vol.,

Table 3. Acute neurological disorders affecting the hippocampus

Etiology	Image findings	Clinical presentation	MRI characteristics
Seizure		unspecific symptoms (altered vigilance, confusion, alterations in mental status, aphasia, hemiparesis); single seizure (febrile, psychomotor, generalized tonic-clonic); repetitive seizures and status epileticus (non-convulsive, focal convulsive, complex partial, generalized tonic-clonic)	DWI involvement of the lateral hippocampus; additional DWI hyperintensity in the pulvinar or the cortex; ADC reduced; frequently accompanied by signs of hyperperfusion
TGA		sudden onset of antero- and retrograde amnesia; complete resolution within 24 h; no disturbance of consciousness; no other neurological deficit or features of ictal activity	small circumscribed DWI lesions of 1–2 mm in diameter in lateral part of the hippocampus, CA1 region; ADC reduced; delayed occurrence
Encephalitis (HSV, HHV, limbic encephalitis)		subacute onset of altered vigilance, confusion; memory deficits and psychiatric symptoms; seizures	DWI hyperintensity of uncus, amygdala, hippocampus; with or without ADC reduction; may extend to the extratemporal structures; accompanied by T2 hyperintensity

HSV = Herpes simplex virus; HHV = human herpes virus.

pp. 143–149]). MRI studies have been unable to detect convincing evidence of hippocampal abnormalities in the acute phase of TGA [20]. This finding suggests that mechanisms other than ischemic infarction cause TGA. Using a modified study design to investigate TGA patients with serial DWI measurements performed from the day of symptom onset through days 1 and 2, recent studies have demonstrated small diffusion-weighted MRI hyperintense lesions in the CA1 subfield of the hippocampal cornu ammonis appearing 24–48 h after the TGA episode, thereby linking the disease to the hippocampus [21]. In most cases, the observed lesions corresponded with a small area with reduced signal on ADC maps and a high signal on T2-weighted images. In a large number of published papers on this phenomenon, these lesions have been detected in up to 90% of TGA patients. There are several factors recognized to be crucial for the detection rate:

- The time between onset and MRI: over 80% of patients displayed punctuate hippocampal DWI changes after 24–48 h, but only about 6% of patients in the acute phase.
- Slice thickness of 3 mm or less: a recent study found an increase of lesion detection by 8.4% per mm [22].
- The b value or diffusion-weighting factor: it was reported recently that DWI obtained at higher b values (b = 2,000 or 3,000) has a higher lesion-detection rate than using a conventional b value of 1,000 [23].
- Higher magnetic field strength: a higher detection rate at 3 T versus 1.5 T has been described (80 vs. 57% at 1.5 T) in TGA patients examined within 12–24 h after symptom onset [24].

It is advisable to optimize the sequences used according to the first three factors when examining patients with suspected TGA.

Seizures and Status Epilepticus

The first reports on hippocampal DWI changes in patients with seizures were published at the beginning of this century. Kim et al. [25] presented a case series of patients with generalized tonic-clonic seizures or status epilepticus, and demonstrated increased signal intensity on DWI in the hippocampus in 3 patients and in the parahippocampal gyrus in 1 patient. Another case report described increased DWI signal in the hippocampus, temporoparietal cortex, and cerebellum, and hyperperfusion in the ipsilateral hemisphere in a patient with focal convulsive status epilepticus [26]. In children with new-onset psychomotor seizures, diffusion abnormalities were found in the complete hippocampus. Interestingly, all of them developed hippocampal atrophy as detected on follow-up MRI and continued to have occasional seizures or developed even intractable complex partial epilepsy [27]. In 2005, a case series of patients with symptomatic complex partial status epilepticus and diffusion abnormalities was published that showed hippocampal hyperintensity in 8 out of 10 patients [28]. The most frequent location of these findings was the hippocampal formation together with the pulvinar region of the thalamus, whereas isolated involvement of the hippocampal formation or of cortical regions occurred less often. Matching areas of decreased ADC signals were found in all cases as well as slight focal swelling accompanied by hyperintensity on T2-weighted images. In contrast to these findings, Di Bonaventura et al. [29] found hippocampal diffusion changes in only 2 out of 10 patients with complex partial status epilepticus although DWI revealed signal alterations in all patients. Similarly, these signal changes resolved completely before the follow-up MRI. A series of 54 patients demonstrated heterogeneity of the phenomenon of peri-ictal DWI changes after status epilepticus and showed that these signal changes are closely related to ipsilateral EEG abnormalities [30].

The pathogenesis of these DWI abnormalities in seizures and status epilepticus is believed to be a result of compromised energy metabolism as prolonged ictal activity is known to increase glucose utilization, the increase of which is not adequately matched by the enhanced blood flow. Consequently, this imbalance of supply and demand may lead to cytogenic and vasogenic edema resulting in restricted diffusion detected on DWI and ADC. In contrast to acute ischemia, where DWI reveals diffusion abnormalities within 30 min and before any T2 signal changes appear, in ongoing status epilepticus DWI and T2 signal changes may occur simultaneously. This finding probably indicates a different pathophysiology with cytotoxic edema induced by the ictal activity preceding a manifest energy deficiency. In turn, this might explain the frequently observed reversibility of DWI changes in patients with seizures or status epilepticus [28, 31].

Infections and Inflammatory Diseases

The most common inflammatory disease affecting the hippocampus is limbic encephalitis that occurs in three major forms: (1) a paraneoplastic subtype which is related to onconeural antibodies in patients with malignant tumors, (2) a nonparaneoplastic subtype that is caused mainly by voltage-gated potassium channel antibodies, and (3) an infectious subtype caused by the herpes virus. The clinical presentation is characterized by a subacute onset of seizures, memory deficits, confusional state, altered vigilance, and psychiatric symptoms.

In paraneoplastic and nonparaneoplastic limbic encephalitis, only a few case reports [32, 33] and a single case series [34] demonstrated hippocampal DWI abnormalities and it remained unclear whether these represented cytotoxic edema or just a T2 shine-through effect. Limbic encephalitis has also been increasingly recognized as a typical finding in immune-compromised patients, in particular after allogeneic hematopoietic stem cell transplantation in hematologic malignancies. The clinical presentation is not different to that observed in paraneoplastic or nonparaneoplastic limbic encephalitis. It is caused by human herpes virus-6, a ubiquitous neurotropic DNA virus known to cause exanthema subitum and sometimes febrile seizures in childhood and to persist lifelong in about 90% of adults. The first case reports on hippocampal DWI hyperintensities in human herpes virus-6 encephalitis were published in 2006 [35, 36]. While in the first report the ADC was reduced in only one patient considered by the authors as a consequence of recent seizures, the authors of the latter discussed cytotoxic edema as a substantial part in the acute pathology of human herpes virus-6 encephalitis. In a more comprehensive case series, Seeley et al. [37] described clinical and MRI findings in 8 patients with human herpes virus-6 encephalitis. All patients demonstrated hyperintensities within the uncus, amygdala, and hippocampus extending to the entorhinal cortex and subiculum on DWI. However, ADC maps (available in 4 patients) suggested impaired diffusion in only one patient and a T2 shine-through effect in the remaining cases. In comparison to the widespread DWI abnormalities in herpes simplex virus encephalitis including the hippocampal formation and amygdala but also other brain regions such as the insular, frontal, temporal or parietooccipital cortices, increased DWI signal intensity is limited to the hippocampus and amygdala in patients with human herpes virus-6 encephalitis. With regard to the lesion characteristics during the clinical course with an increased DWI signal and reduced ADC values in the early and middle phase (0–30 days after onset) and disappearance of these changes in the late phase (more than 30 days after onset), there were no significant differences between both conditions [38].

Anoxic Encephalopathy and Encephalopathies of Other Etiology

Diffusion abnormalities in different brain regions – including the hippocampus – may also be present in patients with anoxic encephalopathy that can be subdivided into hypoxic-ischemic encephalopathy (e.g. caused by cardiac arrest), hypoxic hypoxia (e.g. caused by suicide by hanging), histotoxic hypoxia (e.g. caused by carbon monoxide poisoning), and anemic hypoxia according to its pathophysiology [39–41].

References

1 de Leon MJ, Golomb J, George AE, Convit A, Tarshish CY, McRae T, De Santi S, Smith G, Ferris SH, Noz M, et al: The radiologic prediction of Alzheimer disease: the atrophic hippocampal formation. AJNR Am J Neuroradiol 1993;14:897–906.

2 Maller JJ, Reglade-Meslin C, Chan P, Daskalakis ZJ, Thomson RH, Anstey KJ, Budge M, Sachdev P, Fitzgerald PB: Hippocampal sulcal cavities: prevalence, risk factors and relationship to memory impairment. Brain Res 2011;1368:222–230.

3 Li Y, Li J, Segal S, Wegiel J, De Santi S, Zhan J, de Leon MJ: Hippocampal cerebrospinal fluid spaces on MR imaging: relationship to aging and Alzheimer disease. AJNR Am J Neuroradiol 2006;27:912–918.

4 Bronen RA, Cheung G: MRI of the normal hippocampus. Magn Reson Imaging 1991;9:497–500.

5 Giorgio A, De Stefano N: Clinical use of brain volumetry. J Magn Reson Imaging 2013;37:1–14.

6 Geuze E, Vermetten E, Bremner JD: MR-based in vivo hippocampal volumetrics: 2. Findings in neuropsychiatric disorders. Mol Psychiatry 2005;10:160–184.

7 Jack CR Jr, Theodore WH, Cook M, McCarthy G: MRI-based hippocampal volumetrics: data acquisition, normal ranges, and optimal protocol. Magn Reson Imaging 1995;13:1057–1064.

8 Boccardi M, Ganzola R, Bocchetta M, Pievani M, Redolfi A, Bartzokis G, Camicioli R, Csernansky J, de Leon M, de Toledo-Morrell L, Killiany R, Lehéricy S, Pantel J, Pruessner J, Soininen H, Watson C, Duchesne S, Jack CJ, Frisoni G: Survey of protocols for the manual segmentation of the hippocampus: preparatory steps towards a joint EADC-ADNI harmonized protocol. J Alzheimers Dis 2011;26:61–75.

9 Malmgren K, Thom M: Hippocampal sclerosis – origins and imaging. Epilepsia 2012;53(suppl 4):19–33.

10 Jackson GD, Berkovic SF, Tress BM, Kalnins RM, Fabinyi GC, Bladin PF: Hippocampal sclerosis can be reliably detected by magnetic resonance imaging. Neurology 1990;40:1869–1875.

11 Moran NF, Lemieux L, Kitchen ND, Fish DR, Shorvon SD: Extrahippocampal temporal lobe atrophy in temporal lobe epilepsy and mesial temporal sclerosis. Brain 2001;124:167–175.

12 Jackson GD, Berkovic SF, Duncan JS, Connelly A: Optimizing the diagnosis of hippocampal sclerosis using MR imaging. AJNR Am J Neuroradiol 1993; 14:753–762.

13 Hofman PA, Fitt G, Mitchell LA, Jackson GD: Hippocampal sclerosis and a second focal lesion – how often is it ipsilateral? Epilepsia 2011;52:718–721.

14 Scheltens P, Leys D, Barkhof F, Huglo D, Weinstein HC, Vermersch P, Kuiper M, Steinling M, Wolters EC, Valk J: Atrophy of medial temporal lobes on MRI in 'probable' Alzheimer's disease and normal ageing: diagnostic value and neuropsychological correlates. J Neurol Neurosurg Psychiatry 1992;55: 967–972.

15 Wahlund LO, Barkhof F, Fazekas F, Bronge L, Augustin M, Sjogren M, Wallin A, Ader H, Leys D, Pantoni L, Pasquier F, Erkinjuntti T, Scheltens P: A new rating scale for age-related white matter changes applicable to MRI and CT. Stroke 2001;32:1318–1322.

16 Cavallin L, Loken K, Engedal K, Oksengard AR, Wahlund LO, Bronge L, Axelsson R: Overtime reliability of medial temporal lobe atrophy rating in a clinical setting. Acta Radiol 2012;53:318–323.

17 Galton CJ, Gomez-Anson B, Antoun N, Scheltens P, Patterson K, Graves M, Sahakian BJ, Hodges JR: Temporal lobe rating scale: application to Alzheimer's disease and frontotemporal dementia. J Neurol Neurosurg Psychiatry 2001;70:165–173.

18 Jack CR Jr, Slomkowski M, Gracon S, Hoover TM, Felmlee JP, Stewart K, Xu Y, Shiung M, O'Brien PC, Cha R, Knopman D, Petersen RC: MRI as a biomarker of disease progression in a therapeutic trial of milameline for AD. Neurology 2003;60:253–260.

19 Gass A, Niendorf T, Hirsch JG: Acute and chronic changes of the apparent diffusion coefficient in neurological disorders – biophysical mechanisms and possible underlying histopathology. J Neurol Sci 2001;186(suppl 1):S15–S23.

20 Gass A, Gaa J, Hirsch J, Schwartz A, Hennerici MG: Lack of evidence of acute ischemic tissue change in transient global amnesia on single-shot echo-planar diffusion-weighted MRI. Stroke 1999;30:2070–2072.

21 Sedlaczek O, Hirsch JG, Grips E, Peters CN, Gass A, Wohrle J, Hennerici M: Detection of delayed focal MR changes in the lateral hippocampus in transient global amnesia. Neurology 2004;62:2165–2170.

22 Scheel M, Malkowsky C, Klingebiel R, Schreiber SJ, Bohner G: Magnetic resonance imaging in transient global amnesia: lessons learned from 198 cases. Clin Neuroradiol 2012;22:335–340.

23 Weon YC, Kim JH, Lee JS, Kim SY: Optimal diffusion-weighted imaging protocol for lesion detection in transient global amnesia. AJNR Am J Neuroradiol 2008;29:1324–1328.

24 Ryoo I, Kim JH, Kim S, Choi BS, Jung C, Hwang SI: Lesion detectability on diffusion-weighted imaging in transient global amnesia: the influence of imaging timing and magnetic field strength. Neuroradiology 2012;54:329–334.

25 Kim JA, Chung JI, Yoon PH, Kim DI, Chung TS, Kim EJ, Jeong EK: Transient MR signal changes in patients with generalized tonicoclonic seizure or status epilepticus: periictal diffusion-weighted imaging. AJNR Am J Neuroradiol 2001;22:1149–1160.

26 El-Koussy M, Mathis J, Lovblad KO, Stepper F, Kiefer C, Schroth G: Focal status epilepticus: follow-up by perfusion- and diffusion MRI. Eur Radiol 2002; 12:568–574.

27 Farina L, Bergqvist C, Zimmerman RA, Haselgrove J, Hunter JV, Bilaniuk LT: Acute diffusion abnormalities in the hippocampus of children with new-onset seizures: the development of mesial temporal sclerosis. Neuroradiology 2004;46:251–257.

28 Szabo K, Poepel A, Pohlmann-Eden B, Hirsch J, Back T, Sedlaczek O, Hennerici M, Gass A: Diffusion-weighted and perfusion MRI demonstrates parenchymal changes in complex partial status epilepticus. Brain 2005;128:1369–1376.

29 Di Bonaventura C, Bonini F, Fattouch J, Mari F, Petrucci S, Carni M, Tinelli E, Pantano P, Bastianello S, Maraviglia B, Manfredi M, Prencipe M, Giallonardo AT: Diffusion-weighted magnetic resonance imaging in patients with partial status epilepticus. Epilepsia 2009;50(suppl 1):45–52.

30 Chatzikonstantinou A, Gass A, Forster A, Hennerici MG, Szabo K: Features of acute DWI abnormalities related to status epilepticus. Epilepsy Res 2011;97: 45–51.

31 Parmar H, Lim SH, Tan NC, Lim CC: Acute symptomatic seizures and hippocampus damage: DWI and MRS findings. Neurology 2006;66:1732–1735.

32 Chatzikonstantinou A, Szabo K, Ottomeyer C, Kern R, Hennerici MG: Successive affection of bilateral temporomesial structures in a case of non-paraneoplastic limbic encephalitis demonstrated by serial MRI and FDG-PET. J Neurol 2009;256:1753–1755.

33 Thuerl C, Müller K, Laubenberger J, Volk B, Langer M: MR imaging of autopsy-proved paraneoplastic limbic encephalitis in non-Hodgkin lymphoma. AJNR Am J Neuroradiol 2003;24:507–511.

34 Urbach H, Soeder BM, Jeub M, Klockgether T, Meyer B, Bien CG: Serial MRI of limbic encephalitis. Neuroradiology 2006;48:380–386.

35 Gorniak RJ, Young GS, Wiese DE, Marty FM, Schwartz RB: MR imaging of human herpesvirus-6-associated encephalitis in 4 patients with anterograde amnesia after allogeneic hematopoietic stem-cell transplantation. AJNR Am J Neuroradiol 2006; 27:887–891.

36 Noguchi T, Mihara F, Yoshiura T, Togao O, Atsumi K, Matsuura T, Kuroiwa T, Honda H: MR imaging of human herpesvirus-6 encephalopathy after hematopoietic stem cell transplantation in adults. AJNR Am J Neuroradiol 2006;27:2191–2195.

37 Seeley WW, Marty FM, Holmes TM, Upchurch K, Soiffer RJ, Antin JH, Baden LR, Bromfield EB: Posttransplant acute limbic encephalitis: clinical features and relationship to HHV6. Neurology 2007;69:156–165.

38 Noguchi T, Yoshiura T, Hiwatashi A, Togao O, Yamashita K, Nagao E, Uchino A, Hasuo K, Atsumi K, Matsuura T, Kuroiwa T, Mihara F, Honda H, Kudo S: CT and MRI findings of human herpesvirus 6-associated encephalopathy: comparison with findings of herpes simplex virus encephalitis. AJR Am J Roentgenol 2010;194:754–760.

39 Wijdicks EF, Campeau NG, Miller GM: MR imaging in comatose survivors of cardiac resuscitation. AJNR Am J Neuroradiol 2001;22:1561–1565.

40 Campbell BC, Tu HT, Christensen S, Desmond PM, Levi CR, Bladin CF, Hjort N, Ashkanian M, Solling C, Donnan GA, Davis SM, Ostergaard L, Parsons MW: Assessing response to stroke thrombolysis: validation of 24-hour multimodal magnetic resonance imaging. Arch Neurol 2012;69:46–50.

41 Singhal AB, Topcuoglu MA, Koroshetz WJ: Diffusion MRI in three types of anoxic encephalopathy. J Neurol Sci 2002;196:37–40.

42 Cook MJ, Fish DR, Shorvon SD, Straughan K, Stevens JM: Hippocampal volumetric and morphometric studies in frontal and temporal lobe epilepsy. Brain 1992;115:1001–1015.

43 Jack CR Jr: MRI-based hippocampal volume measurements in epilepsy. Epilepsia 1994;35(suppl 6): S21–S29.

Prof. Dr. Kristina Szabo
Department of Neurology, UniversitätsMedizin Mannheim
Theodor-Kutzer-Ufer 1-3
DE–68167 Mannheim (Germany)
E-Mail szabo@neuro.ma.uni-heidelberg.de

Szabo K, Hennerici MG (eds): The Hippocampus in Clinical Neuroscience.
Front Neurol Neurosci. Basel, Karger, 2014, vol 34, pp 85–94 (DOI: 10.1159/000356427)

Functional MRI Studies of the Hippocampus

Frauke Nees · Sebastian T. Pohlack

Department of Cognitive and Clinical Neuroscience, Central Institute of Mental Health, Medical Faculty
Mannheim, Heidelberg University, Mannheim, Germany

Abstract

Developments in tasks and imaging techniques applied over the last decades have yielded substantial support for the hypothesized role of the hippocampus in mnemonic processes. Human imaging research has now moved on to disentangle the contributions of the different hippocampal subregions and adjacent cortices, so as to bridge the gap between rodent and human data. Besides the importance of such studies for basic research, the investigation of hippocampal (dys)function has clinical relevance for diseases ranging from neurological disorders such as Alzheimer's disease or epilepsy to mental disorders such as schizophrenia or anxiety disorders. So far, most of the present review articles and books about the hippocampus and its functions focus on traditional declarative memory paradigms and 'encoding versus retrieval'. In this chapter we concentrate on a less travelled, but not less important, route concerning the role of the hippocampus in a well-established associative learning (encoding) paradigm: pavlovian fear conditioning. Fear conditioning is hypothesized to model aversive associative learning on a nonpathological level and is further assumed to recruit the same networks that are relevant for anxiety disorders, with the hippocampus being specific for contextual fear conditioning. We highlight the findings in humans by addressing its role in mediating spatial and temporal aspects of a context, involving different kinds of a fear-conditioning procedure (delay vs. trace conditioning), and its role in extinction, both from a theoretical and clinical perspective.

© 2014 S. Karger AG, Basel

Since the first reports of an association between the hippocampus and memory processes, a lot has been discovered about its pivotal role in learning and memory. Naturally, the first positron emission tomography (PET) and functional magnetic resonance imaging (fMRI) studies on memory tried to find evidence for hippocampal activation during memory tasks, but produced only mixed results. However, developments in memory tasks and the imaging techniques applied over the subsequent years yielded substantial support for the hypothesized role of the hippocampus in mnemonic processes. By the end of 2012, PubMed had indexed more than 7,000 articles with 'hippocampus' and 'fMRI' as key words, with an annual (increasing) average of more than 600 publications over the last 5 years.

Research soon went on to disentangle the contributions of different medial temporal lobe (MTL) structures such as the hippocampal region (CA1–3, dentate gyrus, and subiculum) and the adjacent entorhinal, perirhinal, and parahippocampal cortices. Today, our understanding of the MTL system and the role of subcomponents in specific forms of memory is quite advanced based on the study of amnesic patients, electrophysiological recording, and neuroimaging research, with several excellent books and review articles on the latest developments. Imaging data point to a clear role of the hippocampal region in explicit/declarative, but not implicit, memory [Opitz, this vol., pp. 51–59]. In contrast, hippocampal activation could be observed during encoding as well as during retrieval. For the time-limited role of this structure in explicit memory, neuroimaging studies have produced conflicting results. Furthermore, traditional imaging studies do not support a clear functional segregation of the hippocampal region and adjacent structures, and they lack the necessary spatial resolution.

Recent advances in MR physics such as high-resolution (hr) fMRI using smaller and smaller voxel dimensions might enable solutions of such pending problems. Employing hr-fMRI, a reliable segmentation of the hippocampus and parahippocampus based on structural atlases and standards into their respective subcomponents has become feasible allowing the investigation of MTL structures on a more fine-grained level.

Several main research targets have been investigated in this growing field. First, for the differentiation of encoding and retrieval within the hippocampal circuits, earlier studies found a striking dissociation between input (dentate gyrus/CA2–3) and output (CA1 and subiculum) structures: whereas input subfields were selectively active during encoding, activity in the CA1 region and the subiculum was associated with retrieval [1]. However, later studies were unable to reproduce this clear distinction, underlining the need for additional data.

A second core research target for hr-fMRI studies in humans was the association of pattern separation and pattern completion with different hippocampal subfields (e.g. [2]). The terms 'pattern separation' and 'pattern completion' refer to specific processes by which the hippocampus mediates learning and memory. Pattern separation is a process of making similar events or inputs distinct via neural representations which are nonoverlapping in order to reduce memory interference. With the contrasting mechanism, pattern completion, partial cues are mapped to the (more complete or correct) stored conjunctive pattern. While pattern separation is thought to be rooted in the dentate gyrus/CA2–3 hippocampal subfields, pattern completion recruits CA1 and the subiculum (for a review see [3]).

A third line of hr-fMRI research focused on spatial memory using virtual reality paradigms. Here, the authors were able to support rodent data by identifying the CA1 region as the most critical hippocampal subfield for spatial navigation. In sum, hr-fMRI studies offer (despite being technically challenging in nature) a means to study the human hippocampal formation at the individual subfield level, thereby bridging the gap between rodent and human data.

Besides the importance of such studies for basic research, the investigation of hippocampal function and (more so) dysfunction holds obvious clinical relevance for several disorders such as Alzheimer's disease and epilepsy or even planning surgical operations. However, hippocampal impairments also play an important role in several mental disorders such as schizophrenia or anxiety disorders (for a review see [4]). While schizophrenia research has focused on the hippocampal formation for decades, the understanding of the significance of this structure for anxiety disorders such as posttraumatic stress disorder (PTSD) has grown more slowly. Therefore, and since most of the present review articles and books about the hippocampus and its functions focus on the traditional declarative memory paradigms mentioned above, encoding versus retrieval, or the clinical perspective on schizophrenia, the remainder of this chapter will concentrate on a less-travelled route concerning the role of the hippocampus in a well-established associative learning (encoding) paradigm: pavlovian fear conditioning.

Since the first description of classical conditioning by Pavlov in 1927, a large number of studies have used conditioning paradigms to investigate associative learning processes in animal and human research. Additionally, pavlovian fear conditioning has widely been used as a model of anxiety disorders where deficits in fear learning are assumed to play a crucial role in the etiology and maintenance of the disorder [5]. During a typical fear-conditioning paradigm, subjects learn to predict aversive outcomes based on prior experience. In particular, an aversive unconditioned stimulus (US), such as a loud noise or an electric shock, is paired with an initially neutral stimulus (e.g. a geometrical figure or a specific room) and, over time, becomes associated with the aversive event. Hence, the stimulus becomes a conditioned stimulus (CS) which elicits a conditioned reaction comparable to the fearful unconditioned reaction seen after exposure to the US. The majority of studies in animals and humans have used concrete cues, such as a light, tone, or geometrical figures as a CS. When the US is presented without any specific cue, it becomes associated with the context. While conditioned cues evoke phasic fear responses, contexts lead to sustained anxiety responses [6], mimicking specific features of anxiety disorders such as PTSD, panic disorder, or generalized anxiety disorder, which could not be modeled by cued fear-conditioning procedures.

Fear conditioning is hypothesized to model aversive associative learning on a nonpathological level, but is assumed to recruit the same networks that are relevant for anxiety disorders. While cues activate the central nucleus of the amygdala, during contextual fear conditioning the recruitment of the hippocampus is necessary. Compared to the wealth of findings from animal studies, research on the neuronal substrates of contextual fear conditioning in humans remains scarce. The first imaging study comparing cerebral blood flow during cued versus contextual fear conditioning used PET in healthy participants and found distinct networks involved in cued compared to contextual fear conditioning. While the amygdala was only found to be differentially activated during cued fear conditioning, the hippocampus was only recruited during contextual fear conditioning [7]. The first studies using fMRI appeared in short succession

[8–10]. Marschner et al. [10] again used a combined cued and contextual fear-conditioning paradigm. They found a similar dissociation of the amygdala and hippocampus during cued and contextual fear learning which was transient in nature, i.e. activation was rapidly declining. In contrast, Alvarez et al. [8] used a differential contextual fear-conditioning paradigm employing virtual reality without concrete cues. The authors reported activation of the hippocampus as well as the amygdala. The main new feature of the contextual fear-conditioning study by Lang et al. [9] was an extinction phase directly after acquisition. Briefly, hippocampal activity was found during acquisition and a connectivity analysis revealed correlations between the hippocampus and anterior cingulate cortex during acquisition, and the latter regions and the amygdala during extinction. Lastly, a recent study employing cued as well as contextual fear conditioning in a virtual reality paradigm [11] focused on trait anxiety and reported significant involvement of the hippocampus and the ventral prefrontal cortex during contextual fear conditioning. Additionally, the role of the interaction between the two structures was discussed within the framework of emotion regulation prior to extinction.

Since some imaging studies on contextual fear conditioning did not report or observe hippocampal activation and the majority used rather small or selected samples (e.g. males only), we decided to investigate brain activation in a differential contextual fear-conditioning paradigm in a large sample (n = 118) of healthy volunteers [12]. Here we observed robust hippocampal activation during the acquisition, but not during the extinction phase.

In summary, activation of the hippocampus seems to be specific for contextual but not cued fear conditioning, where hippocampal activation is detected in less than 25% of the studies only (for a review see [4]). But what exactly does the hippocampus do during contextual fear learning? The specific role of the hippocampus has been the subject of much debate among animal researchers (where most of our current knowledge comes from) and is now assumed to relate more to mnemonic processes than to performance. While the simple delayed cued fear conditioning relies heavily on the amygdala, where the US-CS association is formed, the role of the hippocampus is most likely in binding together different elements of a context into one figure, which can then be associated with a US in the amygdala [13]. This basic mechanism of the hippocampal circuitry has been termed conjunctive representation. Additionally, another basic hippocampus-dependent mechanism is recruited during contextual fear learning: pattern separation. As could be shown in rodents, posttraining lesions impair contextual memory as long as the internal representation is stored within the hippocampus. Once the memory has been stored independent of the hippocampus, the contextual memory remains intact even after hippocampal ablation, although it may be more general or imprecise. Thus, if the hippocampus is unimpaired, it is responsible for the differentiation between similar but distinct contexts – the latest human research is well in line with these studies [14].

So far, the term 'context' has been used and operationalized in the meaning of a spatial context. However, context encloses not only the spatial dimension, but also the temporal aspect of a given situation. Using another variation of the classical pavlovian approach, namely trace (in contrast to delay) conditioning, the importance of this dimension for hippocampal involvement becomes evident. Derived from research on classical eyeblink conditioning, the differentiation of two associative learning processes, delay and trace conditioning, which differ in the temporal contiguity, i.e. the temporal relationship between the CS and US, and their underlying neural substrates were consistently demonstrated in animals and thus has also become an important tool for investigating learning and memory processes in humans [15]. In delay conditioning the US is presented together with the CS and coterminates with the CS, while in trace conditioning the US and CS are separated by a temporal gap (e.g. 400–700 ms; trace interval). Animal research on classical eyeblink conditioning has consistently shown that specifically two brain regions play an important role in delay versus trace conditioning: the cerebellum and the hippocampus [15]. While the cerebellum is essential for delay eyeblink conditioning, the hippocampus is the central target necessary for normal functioning of associative trace (eyeblink) conditioning mediating the CS-US contingency.

So far, however, most of what we know about the role of the hippocampus during delay versus trace conditioning stems from animal and human lesion studies. Functional imaging studies in humans are rare. A recent work by Cheng et al. [16] combined fMRI during delay and trace eyeblink conditioning by using a within-subject design. Participants watched a silent movie while receiving pseudoconditioning [four blocks of delay-alone, trace-alone, and airpuff (US)-alone] and acquisition blocks (16 alternating delay and trace blocks each). This study supports and extends previous animal work as well as data from human lesion and electrophysiology studies by providing further evidence that the hippocampus is a functional target brain region in trace conditioning. Higher hippocampal responses were found during trace compared to delay eyeblink conditioning. Although the timing of this increased hippocampal response was found to coincide with conditioned responses on a behavioural level in both delay and trace conditioning, it was found even when the behavioural expression of delay and trace conditioned responses were comparable. This indicates that the hippocampus may be critically relied on during trace association rather than being strictly performance related.

These data on the involvement of the hippocampus in eyeblink conditioning provide evidence to assume that such a brief technically simple and noninvasive paradigm might be a useful diagnostic tool for hippocampus-related disorders such as dementia. It allows to differentiate those disorders from normal aging as well as to identify them already at early stages, which is critical for the success of therapeutic strategies. For example, in Alzheimer's disease the earliest pathology occurs in the entorhinal input to the hippocampus. In this case, impaired eyeblink conditioning can be the result of dysfunctions in MTL structures that disrupt input to the cerebellum, and eyeblink conditioning may thus indicate early disruptions before impairments of declarative learning and memory appear [17]. This further supports the assumption that trace conditioning is highly hippocampus-dependent and underlines the need for functional imaging studies on the role of the hippocampus in trace eyeblink conditioning in both healthy humans and individuals with hippocampus-dependent disorders.

From a constructivist point of view, delay (eyeblink) conditioning is considered to represent implicit learning independent of subjective awareness of CS-US contingency, whereas trace (eyeblink) conditioning depends on the contingency awareness and represents a form of explicit learning [18]. As mentioned above, the hippocampus is involved in learning processes, that specifically play a crucial role in contextual modulation. In learning and expression of conditioned responses, contexts are important aspects. While a generalization of conditioned responses across contexts is assumed after acquisition, conditioned responses during or following extinction are context specific (e.g. [19]). Although our understanding of how the brain mediates the effects of context on extinction is still growing, there is already considerable evidence that the hippocampus is involved in contextual representations during fear conditioning and it has subsequently become a target brain region in investigations on the contextual modulation of fear extinction. Also during trace eyeblink conditioning, where individuals have to spend more cognitive effort to bridge the (temporal) gap between the CS and US, a key role of the hippocampus may thus specifically be assumed for context effects (e.g. context shifts) during trace conditioning, especially after extinction.

So far, context dependence of extinction has been demonstrated, for example, using renewal experiments, where conditioned responses occur during exposure to the acquisition context following extinction training in a different context [19]. Interestingly, using a virtual environment in humans, renewal could be demonstrated only in delay, but not trace, eyeblink conditioning [20]. Although there is no clear explanation for this lack of renewal following trace conditioning, it can be assumed that cognitive factors play an important role: higher effort in trace conditioning based on the time interval between CS and US might make this procedure more difficult compared to the delay procedure (implicit vs. explicit memory). The renewal context might gather attention which may interfere with performance through inhibiting trace-conditioned responses by binding attention on external resources [21].

However, how the hippocampus is involved in this process has not yet been evaluated, but would be interesting from more than just a theoretical perspective. Extinction of prior threat-related associations requires new learning and with its relation to contextual influences this process may be more fragile in contrast to the acquisition of conditioned fear responses. Additionally, it is highly important in terms of a clinical perspective, given that such factors are key components to address in the treatment of several disorders, for example anxiety disorders (e.g. [19]). Research on extinction would give further insight into the complex nature of these mechanisms and the specific role of the hippocampus.

So far, previous neuroimaging studies on extinction processes within classical conditioning have implicated not only the hippocampus, but also the amygdala and the ventromedial prefrontal cortex as important structures in extinction recall [22]. In line with findings from animal studies, this neural network is assumed to contribute to the contextual modulation of conditioned responses. However, elucidating the critical role of the hippocampus 'alone' on contextual control of fear extinction, a growing body of research supports the involvement of the hippocampus in context-related encoding and retrieval of extinction memory as well as context-specific regulation of extinction.

For example, in line with animal models (e.g. [19]), it has been shown that the hippocampus plays a role in context modulation of extinction retention in humans by demonstrating an impaired reinstatement of conditioned fear in individuals with hippocampal damage [23]. In reinstatement, few presentations of the US in the extinction context result in recovery of the previously extinguished conditioned response. Data from lesion studies on hippocampal inactivation prior to extinction and dorsal hippocampal inactivation before extinction recall indicate so far that the hippocampus is involved in whether an individual will fall back on recalling fear or extinction memory based on contextual cues in a specific situation [24]. However, functional imaging studies in humans are rare, but to prove this role also in a functional manner would be of great importance for future research (fig. 1).

Moreover, in addition to previous animal data that have elaborated the role of the hippocampus in mediating contextual control of extinction, the few data in humans also provide evidence that the hippocampus mediates context-dependent extinction memory (e.g. [23, 25]). A functional imaging study by Kalisch et al. [25] examined context-dependent retrieval processes and found a higher response in the hippocampus as well as the ventromedial prefrontal cortex after extinction in an extinction-related, but not conditioning-related, context. This finding of a hippocampal-ventromedial prefrontal network involvement in context-dependent recall of extinction memory does not only further support a role of the hippocampus in conferring contextual information, but also underline the importance of the connectivity between different brain regions in extinction. Similar results could be demonstrated in another study that also identified different brain regions during extinction recall in healthy humans using fMRI [22]. Milad et al. [22] used a novel design in which they differentiated extinction recall from conditioning recall. Using a standard differential conditioning design, participants received acquisition and extinction blocks with visual CS presented within photographs of two distinct rooms serving as contexts on day 1. An extinction recall block was implemented on day 2 in which responses to the CS in the extinction context was tested. During extinction recall, significantly increased responses in the hippocampus and ventromedial prefrontal cortex to a previously extinguished compared to an unextinguished CS could be observed. In addition, positive correlations of the magnitude of these brain responses with extinction memory as well as between the neural responses in both brain regions were also reported.

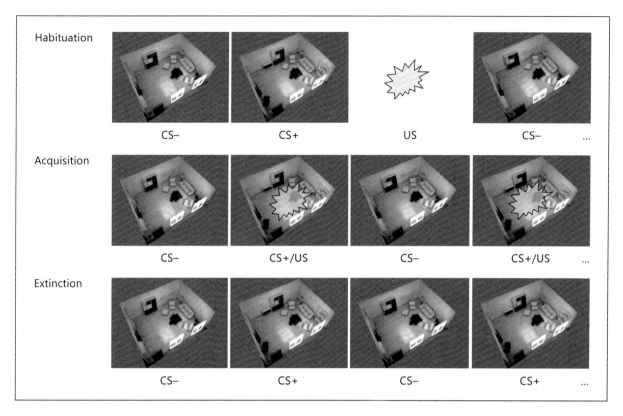

Fig. 1. Example of the experimental setup of a contextual conditioning paradigm: two pictures depict different contexts serving as conditioned stimuli (CS+/−); an aversive scream is used as the unconditioned stimulus (US).

These findings further underline the importance of the hippocampus, together with the ventromedial prefrontal cortex, in the recall of extinction memory.

Deficits in extinction might be important for the development and maintenance of anxiety disorders involving PTSD (e.g. [26]). From a clinical standpoint, fear extinction for example represents the main ingredient of exposure-based therapy. The delineation of the role of the hippocampus in fear extinction advances the understanding of anxiety disorders and provides an important background for therapeutic approaches.

So far, for example, in anxiety disorders context-renewal effects could be demonstrated in exposure therapy [27], and stronger acquisition and retention of fear associations were observed in clinically anxious compared to nonanxious individuals. However, whether anxiety is primarily related to stronger acquisition and/or impaired extinction is still not completely clear. PTSD has been characterized by exaggerated acquisition of fear associations (represented by increased responses in the amygdala), by deficits in fear extinction (represented by dysfunctions in the frontal cortex), and by impairments in the appreciation of safe contexts and explicit learning and memory (represented by dysfunctions in the hippocampus) [26]. It has been shown to be associated with volumetric and functional impairments in the hippocampus, but it is not yet clear if and how dysfunctions in the hippocampus contribute to the development and maintenance of PTSD.

In line with the knowledge gained from animal studies that the hippocampus is involved in building and recalling associations between aversive events and contextual stimuli, but not simple cues, reduced hippocampal function, as described for example in PTSD, can induce the association of multiple cues and increase the occurrence of fear responses in multiple contexts in which these cues are present. This could explain characteristics known from individuals with PTSD such as fear responses to trauma reminders outside of contexts in which these cues would reasonably predict danger [28]. However, as mentioned above, it should be noted that fear extinction and recall are assumed to not only depend on the function of the hippocampus but specifically extinction learning to also rely on the amygdala, and fear inhibition during extinction recall additionally on the ventromedial prefrontal cortex [24]. For the contextual regulation of extinction recall, both animal and human studies have shown a coactivation of the ventromedial prefrontal cortex and hippocampus, whose dysfunction is assumed to be associated with anxiety disorders.

In sum, in the present chapter, we aimed to demonstrate that the function of the hippocampus is not a simple one, but very complex involving factors ranging from external conditions such as temporal relationships to the brain structure itself (pattern separation), and that these complex interferences are differentially expressed in mental and neurological disorders.

Outlook

To date, there have been some interesting discrepancies between findings from animal studies on the role of the hippocampus and theories on hippocampal functions conferring risk to develop anxiety disorders. The hippocampus has been shown to play not only a role in contextual fear conditioning in general, but also in contextual reinstatement of conditioned fear as shown after hippocampal damage, in generalization of extinction across contexts following pharmacological inactivation of the hippocampus, and in renewal of conditioned fear. So far, it has been commonly discussed that the reduced functioning of the hippocampus often observed for example in PTSD might be a risk factor for the development and maintenance of this disorder by limiting the ability to appreciate safe contexts. However, one could also hypothesize that dysfunctions in the hippocampus can be protective by interference with fear conditioning and thus promote the generalization of extinction. Therefore, there might be several ways of how dysfunctions in the hippocampus might influence disorders such as PTSD. Further research is needed to uncover the functional role of the hippocampus in context conditioning and contextual modulation of extinction in more detail.

References

1 Eldridge LL, Engel SA, Zeineh MM, Bookheimer SY, Knowlton BJ: A dissociation of encoding and retrieval processes in the human hippocampus. J Neurosci 2005;25:3280–3286.

2 Bakker A, Kirwan CB, Miller M, Stark CE: Pattern separation in the human hippocampal CA3 and dentate gyrus. Science 2008;319:1640–1642.

3 Carr VA, Rissman J, Wagner AD: Imaging the human medial temporal lobe with high-resolution fMRI. Neuron 2010;65:298–308.

4 Sehlmeyer C, Schoning S, Zwitserlood P, Pfleiderer B, Kircher T, Arolt V, et al: Human fear conditioning and extinction in neuroimaging: a systematic review. PLoS One 2009;4:e5865.

5 Mineka S, Oehlberg K: The relevance of recent developments in classical conditioning to understanding the etiology and maintenance of anxiety disorders. Acta Psychol (Amst) 2008;127:567–580.

6 Marks IM: Fears, Phobias, and Rituals: Panic, Anxiety, and Their Disorders. New York, Oxford University Press, 1987.

7 Hasler G, Fromm S, Alvarez RP, Luckenbaugh DA, Drevets WC, Grillon C: Cerebral blood flow in immediate and sustained anxiety. J Neurosci 2007;27:6313–6319.

8 Alvarez RP, Biggs A, Chen G, Pine DS, Grillon C: Contextual fear conditioning in humans: cortical-hippocampal and amygdala contributions. J Neurosci 2008;28:6211–6219.

9 Lang S, Kroll A, Lipinski SJ, Wessa M, Ridder S, Christmann C, et al: Context conditioning and extinction in humans: differential contribution of the hippocampus, amygdala and prefrontal cortex. Eur J Neurosci 2009;29:823–832.

10 Marschner A, Kalisch R, Vervliet B, Vansteenwegen D, Buchel C: Dissociable roles for the hippocampus and the amygdala in human cued versus context fear conditioning. J Neurosci 2008;28:9030–9036.

11 Indovina I, Robbins TW, Nunez-Elizalde AO, Dunn BD, Bishop SJ: Fear-conditioning mechanisms associated with trait vulnerability to anxiety in humans. Neuron 2011;69:563–571.

12 Pohlack ST, Nees F, Ruttorf M, Schad LR, Flor H: Activation of the ventral striatum during aversive contextual conditioning in humans. Biol Psychol 2012;91:74–80.

13 Maren S: Neurobiology of Pavlovian fear conditioning. Annu Rev Neurosci 2001;24:897–931.

14 Olsen RK, Moses SN, Riggs L, Ryan JD: The hippocampus supports multiple cognitive processes through relational binding and comparison. Front Hum Neurosci 2012;6:146.

15 Christian KM, Thompson RF: Neural substrates of eyeblink conditioning: acquisition and retention. Learn Mem 2003;10:427–455.

16 Cheng DT, Disterhoft JF, Power JM, Ellis DA, Desmond JE: Neural substrates underlying human delay and trace eyeblink conditioning. Proc Natl Acad Sci USA 2008;105:8108–8113.

17 Woodruff-Pak DS: Eyeblink classical conditioning differentiates normal aging from Alzheimer's disease. Integr Physiol Behav Sci 2001;36:87–108.

18 Clark RE, Squire LR: Classical conditioning and brain systems: the role of awareness. Science 1998;280:77–81.

19 Bouton ME: Context and behavioral processes in extinction. Learn Mem 2004;11:485–494.

20 Grillon C, Alvarez RP, Johnson L, Chavis C: Contextual specificity of extinction of delay but not trace eyeblink conditioning in humans. Learn Mem 2008;15:387–389.

21 Clark CR, Squire LR: Human eyeblink classical conditioning: effects of manipulating awareness of the stimulus contingencies. Psychol Sci 1999;10:14–18.

22 Milad MR, Wright CI, Orr SP, Pitman RK, Quirk GJ, Rauch SL: Recall of fear extinction in humans activates the ventromedial prefrontal cortex and hippocampus in concert. Biol Psychiatry 2007;62:446–454.

23 LaBar KS, Phelps EA: Reinstatement of conditioned fear in humans is context dependent and impaired in amnesia. Behav Neurosci 2005;119:677–686.

24 Corcoran KA, Quirk GJ: Recalling safety: cooperative functions of the ventromedial prefrontal cortex and the hippocampus in extinction. CNS Spectr 2007;12:200–206.

25 Kalisch R, Korenfeld E, Stephan KE, Weiskopf N, Seymour B, Dolan RJ: Context-dependent human extinction memory is mediated by a ventromedial prefrontal and hippocampal network. J Neurosci 2006;26:9503–9511.

26 Rauch SL, Shin LM, Phelps EA: Neurocircuitry models of posttraumatic stress disorder and extinction: human neuroimaging research – past, present, and future. Biol Psychiatry 2006;60:376–382.

27 Hermans D, Craske MG, Mineka S, Lovibond PF: Extinction in human fear conditioning. Biol Psychiatry 2006;60:361–368.

28 Acheson DT, Gresack JE, Risbrough VB: Hippocampal dysfunction effects on context memory: possible etiology for posttraumatic stress disorder. Neuropharmacology 2012;62:674–685.

Frauke Nees, PhD
Department of Cognitive and Clinical Neuroscience
Central Institute of Mental Health, Square J 5
DE–68159 Mannheim (Germany)
E-Mail frauke.nees@zi-mannheim.de

Szabo K, Hennerici MG (eds): The Hippocampus in Clinical Neuroscience.
Front Neurol Neurosci. Basel, Karger, 2014, vol 34, pp 95–108 (DOI: 10.1159/000356430)

The Hippocampus in Neurodegenerative Disease

K.K. Moodley · D. Chan

Brighton and Sussex Medical School, Brighton, UK

Abstract

AD is the commonest neurodegenerative disorder resulting ultimately in dementia, a stage during which there is a loss of previously acquired intellectual skill and independent occupational and social function. Neurodegenerative changes within the hippocampus and an extended neuronal network involving the medial temporal and medial parietal lobe result in the archetypal memory impairment seen in Alzheimer's disease (AD). As attention focuses increasingly on early diagnosis and treatment of dementia, this understanding of the hippocampal involvement in AD has helped to develop diagnostic tools for use in early disease. However, hippocampal damage is also a common feature among non-AD neurodegenerative dementias. Neuroimaging techniques, in conjunction with behavioral and pathological techniques, can be used to determine the involvement of the hippocampus in AD and other neurodegenerative diseases.   © 2014 S. Karger AG, Basel

Alzheimer's Disease

Alzheimer's disease (AD) is a progressive neurodegenerative disorder that is typically manifest in the eighth decade of life, presenting initially with an insidious memory disturbance that heralds progressive cognitive and functional decline and culminating in dementia. AD is the commonest cause of dementia, affecting over 36 million people worldwide associated with an estimated healthcare expenditure in excess of USD 600 billion. The World Health Organization has identified dementia due to AD as a public health priority that, without an effective preventative strategy, will impact an estimated 115 million people worldwide by 2050.

The neuropathological cascade that underpins AD neurodegeneration is now understood to begin decades before the emergence of cognitive decline, such that the phase of the disease characterized by the development of dementia represents the final phase of AD. The incidence of AD rises with age, doubling every 5 years after the age of 65, with the disease being present in over a quarter of those greater than 85 years of age.

Alzheimer's Disease Pathophysiology
On macroscopic examination, AD brains are associated with brain atrophy, manifest as widening of cerebral sulci and ventricular dilatation. Atrophy is most marked in the medial temporal lobe (MTL) with initial changes in the entorhinal cortex (EC) and subsequently the hippocampus [1].

Microscopically, extracellular amyloid plaques and intracellular neurofibrillary tangles (NFTs), first identified by Alois Alzheimer in 1907, are the hallmark histopathological features of disease. While the exact mechanisms that link amyloid and tau remain to be elucidated, there is substantial evidence supporting their involvement in the widespread synaptic loss and cerebral hypometabolism that precedes overt neuronal losses in AD.

Amyloid
Amyloid plaques in AD exists in two forms: diffuse plaques that largely only contain aggregated extracellular β-amyloid peptide (Aβ), and neuritic plaques (NPs) that are more compact containing a core of Aβ aggregated with apolipoprotein E, complement, and degenerating neuronal and glial processes.

Aβ is produced under physiological conditions by the sequential cleavage of the amyloid precursor protein (APP), a glycoprotein usually located on cell, endoplasmic reticulum, and mitochondrial membranes. In AD, the homeostatic control of Aβ production and removal is impaired resulting in the accumulation of Aβ 1–42, a particularly oligomeric isomer of Aβ leading in turn to the generation of neurotoxic dimers and other oligomers. Soluble Aβ oligomers are detectable within the pyramidal neurons of the EC and the CA1 hippocampal subfield from the earliest stages of AD and are associated with endosomal enlargement, impaired mitochondrial function, and decreased synaptic and dendritic spine density [2]. Experimental work involving the Tg2576 transgenic mouse model of AD has also shown that brain levels of a particular Aβ dodecamer, Aβ*56, is correlated with spatial memory impairment, while human study suggests that Aβ*56 is overexpressed in ageing and correlates with the presence of soluble tau pathology, the absence of postsynaptic proteins, and cognitive impairment [3].

The extracellular deposition of Aβ is first detectable in the dorsolateral neocortex (posterior then anterior), then the EC and CA1 before involving the remaining MTL and basal forebrain [4]. The polymerization of Aβ 1–42 ultimately results in the formation of protofibrils and insoluble fibrils that aggregate as NPs.

While neocortical NP pathology does not correlate with cognitive impairment, study of the Tg2576 mouse indicates that hippocampal plaque burden in ageing is correlated with impaired place cell firing and spatial memory deficits [5]. In humans, CA1 and the molecular layer of the dentate gyrus appear particularly vulnerable to early NP aggregation associated with altered synaptic density within the perforant path [6], possibly reflecting the sensitivity of CA1 to microglial mediated neuroinflammation in response to NP pathology.

Tau

In AD, dysregulation of phosphokinase activity results in hyperphosphorylation of microtubule-associated tau. This is turn becomes fibrillar forming pretangles, paired helical filaments, and NFTs that accumulate within the perikarya and dendrites of the EC. Experimental work has shown that these conformational changes may facilitate the 'prion-like' spread of NFTs between neurons [7], which may account for the sequential spread of NFT pathology in AD. In Braak stages 1 and 2, pathology is restricted to the EC, appearing to spread in a laminar network that follows the perforant path to involve CA1, spreading to the remaining hippocampal subregions and MTL (stages 3 and 4) and then the neocortex (posterior then anterior, stages 5 and 6) [8]. Tau hyperphosphorylation impairs axonal trafficking that, together with colocalized oligomeric Aβ, functionally disconnects the perforant path [6]. In addition, the distribution and density of NFTs are closely linked to eventual neuronal loss and levels of cognitive impairment such that Braak staging is tightly correlated with clinical dementia severity [9].

Neurotransmitter Alterations: Acetylcholine and N-Methyl-D-Aspartate

The neocortex and amygdala principally derive their cholinergic input from the basal nucleus of Meynert, which is in turn regulated by afferents that relay via the EC and hippocampus. During Braak stages 3 and 4, NFTs and NPs colocalize in the basal nucleus of Meynert, the medial septal nucleus, and the diagonal band, the latter two nuclei representing major sources of acetylcholine to the hippocampus. In AD, the resulting neocortical and allocortical cholinergic deficiency contributes to impairments of complex attention, learning, and memory.

Glutamate-mediated phasic excitation of N-methyl-D-aspartate receptors in the EC and hippocampus is required for place cell functioning, long-term potentiation, and synaptic neuroplasticity. In AD the tonic overactivation of N-methyl-D-aspartate receptors, thought to result from oligomeric Aβ-induced oxidative stress, leads to neurotoxic intracellular calcium accumulation predisposing to cell death.

Understanding these neurotransmitter alterations has led to the use of cholinesterase inhibitors and N-methyl-D-aspartate receptor antagonists to slow down cognitive decline in AD with modest benefit for the former in early dementia and the latter in advanced dementia.

Genetics of Alzheimer's Disease

After advancing age, family history is the second largest risk factor for AD. While the vast majority of AD is late-onset (arbitrarily defined as onset after 65 years), appearing sporadic, more than 50% of the susceptibility for AD is linked to non-Mendelian polymorphisms that interact with age, sex, and vascular risk.

The ε4 allele of the Apolipoprotein E gene (*APOE*, 19q) is the single most significant genetic risk factor for late-onset AD. ε4 homozygotes are 12 times more likely to develop AD compared to noncarriers and are also at risk for an earlier onset of dementia compared to ε4 heterozygotes (in whom the risk of AD is increased threefold compared to noncarriers). In contrast, the ε2 allele appears to be protective against AD. Genetic factors also influence phenotypic aspects of disease: in the case of *APOE,* ε4 is more often associated with accelerated hippocampal atrophy and memory impairment.

Although the effect of other polymorphisms, as identified by genome-wide association studies, are modest at best, these do provide some insights into pathogenesis. For instance, alterations in lipid metabolism (e.g. polymorphisms in *APOE, CLU* and *PICALM*) and cell membrane homeostasis (e.g. *SORL1* and *BIN1*) are implicated in impaired AB neurovascular clearance while immune activation (e.g. *CR1, CD33* and *TREM2*) is implicated in neurotoxicity. This complex genetic heterogeneity may explain the higher than expected incidence of AD in patients with vascular risk factors (insulin resistance, diabetes, hyperhomocysteinemia, smoking, and sedentary lifestyle).

Only 1% of AD is due to fully penetrant autosomal dominant inheritance. Mutations in the *Presenilin 1* (*PSEN1*; located on chromosome 14*)*, *Presenilin 2* (*PSEN2*; chromosome 1), and *APP* (chromosome 21) all result in gene products that are involved in APP processing [10]. The overproduction of Aβ both as a result of these mutations and the triplication of the *APP* gene in Down syndrome is central to the formulation of the 'amyloid hypothesis' of AD [11], which proposes a causal link between Aβ accumulation and AD pathogenesis. While these mutations tend to be associated with an earlier onset of dementia, the description of an autosomal dominant *APP* mutation associated with decreased Aβ 1–42 production and a reduced risk for both AD and age-related memory impairment further suggests that soluble amyloid species are relevant to the development of cognitive impairment [12].

Clinical Presentation
Recently updated clinical and research criteria redefine AD as a disorder with prodromal cognitive and behavioral changes occurring in advance dementia [13, 14].

Dementia due to Alzheimer's Disease
The cardinal symptom of AD is impairment of episodic memory. The symptoms of 'getting lost' and becoming disorientated in time and place are other characteristic features of early AD. Patients may not be aware of the extent of their symptoms due to impaired insight.

The clinical criteria for AD dementia [14] stipulate the need for the progressive impairment of at least two cognitive functions severe enough to cause a loss in social or occupational functioning. These include: aphasia (disturbance of speech and language), apraxia (defective voluntary movements due to disrupted cortical sensorimotor integration), agnosia (impaired object recognition), and impaired executive function (impaired problem-solving, abstract reasoning, and organizational abilities). Clinical AD dementia may be subdivided into mild, moderate, and severe stages based on the degree of cognitive and functional impairment.

While the majority of AD presents with a typical profile of early memory loss and disorientation, there are three recognized atypical variants associated with focal cortical symptoms that precede memory impairment:

- Language presentation (logopenic progressive aphasia): prominent deficits in word finding accompanied by clinical evidence of impaired auditory working memory
- Visuospatial presentation (posterior cortical atrophy): prominent deficits in higher visual processing
- Executive presentation (frontal variant of AD): prominent deficits related to reasoning, abstract thinking and problem solving

Mild Cognitive Impairment due to Alzheimer's Disease

Mild cognitive impairment (MCI) is defined as a symptomatic change in cognitive ability (recognized either by the patient or a third party familiar to the patient) accompanied by measurable cognitive deficits accompanied by retained social and occupational independence.

MCI was originally proposed as a transitional stage between normal ageing and dementia. While MCI conveys an estimated 5–10% annual risk of conversion to AD, different rates of conversion observed in community and hospital clinical cohorts and a proportion of patients remain stable or experience improvement in their symptoms. In view of this heterogeneity in the natural history of MCI as defined on clinical grounds alone, newly issued research criteria [13] define MCI due to AD in terms of the presence of biological markers that indicate underlying AD neuropathology (biomarkers). These include cerebrospinal fluid analysis (decreased Aβ 1–42, increased tau, and increased phosphorylated tau) or neuroimaging markers of disease. As such, MCI in the presence of AD biomarkers has been termed prodromal AD [15].

Presymptomatic Alzheimer's Disease

Presymptomatic AD refers to the clinical stage of the disease that predates the onset of MCI or mild dementia. Study of presymptomatic familial AD cases (the DIAN study) has shown that biomarker evidence of AD and neuroimaging changes predate the onset of cognitive impairment by up to 20 years [16].

Cognitive Changes in Alzheimer's Disease

Memory Impairment

Episodic Memory. Impairment of episodic memory in AD is exemplified by the inability to learn and remember new information and to recall recent events. This is often characterized by poor recollection of recent events, repetitive questioning, and the inability to keep track of appointments and medications accompanied by an increasing dependence on memory supplements such as diaries. Clinically, testing delayed recall serves as a useful test of episodic memory, measuring the ability to register and retrieve either verbal (e.g. a word list) or nonverbal (e.g. design copy) information that must be recalled after a delay spanning minutes. In addition to free recall, respondents can be provided with contextual clues (cueing). Patients with AD perform poorly on these tests and show little response to cueing.

Topographical Memory. Another early symptom of AD is 'getting lost', which initially happens in unfamiliar places, but subsequently also in familiar environments. The hippocampus, particularly the right hippocampus, and the retrosplenial cortex form part of a navigational network that subserves topographical memory. Patients with AD perform poorly on virtual reality navigation tasks [17] and on tasks of topographical working memory involving the recall of visual scenes [18].

Autobiographical Memory. In AD, there is loss of recent autobiographical memory with apparent relative preservation of memory for remote events. However, even within remote memory, it is the content of memory that is preferentially spared with greater impairment noted in the ability to recall the context of an event. These deficits are thought to be due to hippocampal impairment preventing the consolidation of recent autobiographical experiences, but may also indicate that the hippocampus is required for the recall of context related to distant events.

Semantic Memory. The impairment of semantic memory in mild AD is manifest as an inability to generate a word list bound by semantic rules (e.g. names of animals) as opposed to lexical rules (e.g. words starting with a predefined letter of the alphabet), or as a deficit in confrontational naming (for instance when shown a picture array) accompanied by category-specific word errors. In later AD there is loss of general semantic memory such that they develop deficits in generating verbal definitions and naming high-frequency items (e.g. wristwatch), and have impaired comprehension due to loss of word meaning.

Procedural Memory. Procedural memory is typically spared until the advanced stages of disease, reflecting the relative preservation of neostriatal and cerebellar function. Even at a moderate-severe stage of dementia, patients are able to learn a new motor skill although the coexistence of apraxia and agnosia in very advanced disease may prevent a patient from being able to complete even overfamiliar tasks such as shaving or making a cup of tea.

Nonmemory Cognitive Impairment in Alzheimer's Disease

Speech and Language. Word-finding difficulties occur early in AD accompanied by word pauses and compensatory circumlocution. Naming is initially preserved, but the inability to name parts of an object is characteristic of early AD. With disease progression, speech becomes increasingly devoid of grammar and syntax and may become paraphasic accompanied by impaired comprehension. In severe AD, speech may become reiterative, perseverative, or unintelligible due to phonologic deficits. Ultimately, patients may become completely mute.

Apraxia. Apraxia is usually observed at a mild-moderate stage of AD and becomes more severe as the disease progresses. 'Body part as object' errors are particularly common on pantomiming of transitive movements, i.e. when asked to pantomime the use of an imaginary tool, the patient simulates the task using the body part instead of miming the use of the tool. Constructional apraxia is another characteristic feature that may manifest as the inability to copy a complex geometric shape. Ideational apraxia (the knowledge of the action rather than the use of a tool) is also seen in AD and usually reflects further breakdown of semantic function.

Higher Visual Function. Visual agnosia in AD is a disorder of higher visual processing that manifests as impairment objection recognition. This may be apperceptive in nature, due to an inability to perceive objects, or associative, due to an impairment in associating semantic information with the visual percept. Specific forms of agnosia include prosopagnosia, the inability to recognize familiar faces associated with damage to the right temporal lobe, and landmark agnosia, the inability to recognize landmarks (e.g. buildings, monuments, intersections, etc.).

Executive Function. Dysexecutive syndrome is characterized by impaired problem solving, abstract reasoning, and task-switching. It is consistently an early feature of AD and is detectable even in the prodromal phase of illness. During the mild stages of dementia, further deficits in sustained and divided attention become apparent.

Neuropsychiatric Symptoms. Up to 80% of patients with dementia develop neuropsychiatric symptoms. Depression and anxiety are earlier features with agitation, delusions, and paranoia being more common in moderate disease. The latter stages of dementia may be associated with increasing restlessness and wandering.

Clinical Assessment

The physical examination in early AD is often normal. Some patients with familial AD may have abnormal physical signs such as myoclonus or spasticity. In severe AD, patients may develop extrapyramidal signs and other examination abnormalities such as abulia and motor stereotypy.

Cognitive testing varies in different clinical settings but a routine bedside assessment should include at least a screen of executive function, orientation in place and time, episodic memory language, and higher visual processing. The Mini-Mental State Examination (MMSE) [19] is the most widely used screening test for dementia. The major limitations of the MMSE are that it does not measure executive function and that it lacks diagnostic sensitivity and specificity. Other tests like the Addenbrooke's Cognitive Examination (ACE-R) [20] are more comprehensive, providing additional information about language, verbal fluency, and visuoperceptive function that may be useful in discriminating between AD and non-AD dementias.

Neuroimaging

The changes in brain structure and brain function that occur in AD can be detected using a variety of neuroimaging modalities.

Structural Imaging

Structural imaging, using either CT or MRI, is used to determine the topography of brain atrophy in AD.

While CT is clinically useful in excluding nondegenerative causes of cognitive impairment such as tumors and other space-occupying lesions, MRI offers superior spatial resolution. In clinical practice, MRI scans are assessed qualitatively using visual inspection, but MRI measures of MTL atrophy may also be evaluated using semiquantitative techniques, with the 5-point visual rating scale of MTL atrophy being 85% sensitive and 88% specific in distinguishing AD from controls [21].

In research settings, automated methods for analyzing atrophy offers the advantage of both cross-sectional and longitudinal study with the patient acting as their own control, allowing for the detection of progressive atrophy within an individual [21]. Currently employed automated methods include voxel-based morphometry and FreeSurfer, used also to measure cortical thickness.

In AD, longitudinal study has shown a progression of atrophy that bears similarity with the pathological spread of NFTs in the Braak staging system. Atrophy is detected first in the EC followed by the hippocampus, amygdala, and parahippocampus, then spreads to the posterior cingulate gyrus and polymodal association areas, sparing the occipital cortex until late in disease.

Progressive EC volume loss does not appear to be a feature of normal aging, and EC atrophy is both sensitive and specific for AD. However, the anatomical delineation of the EC using MRI is labor intensive as a result of the heterogeneous EC morphology in humans, and poor interrater reliability limits the usage of EC measurements in practice.

By contrast, hippocampal anatomy is easier to segment with corresponding higher measurement reproducibility indices (fig. 1). Longitudinal studies have found that hippocampal atrophy rates in AD are much higher than age-matched controls [22]. The rate of hippocampal atrophy is highest earliest in disease [23], while cortical atrophy rates accelerate later in disease but in advance of correlative cognitive changes. In addition, longitudinal MRI measures can predict the conversion of MCI to AD and is useful in identifying asymptomatic elders at risk for dementia [22]. Hippocampal atrophy is accepted as a biomarker of sporadic AD.

Functional Imaging: FDG-PET, SPECT, and Functional MRI

FDG-PET measures cerebral metabolism by determining the uptake of a radioactive isotope linked to glucose. Decreased FDG uptake (hypometabolism) within the parietotemporal association cortices and posterior cingulate gyrus is characteristic of early AD, while prefrontal hypometabolism is a feature of advanced AD [24]. The specificity and sensitivity of FDG-PET ranges between 71 and 74% and 84 and 95%, respectively. Longitudinal study has demonstrated the predictive value of FDP-PET for determining the progression of MCI to AD and in differentiating between AD and other neurodegenerative diseases causing dementia.

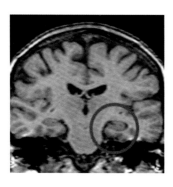
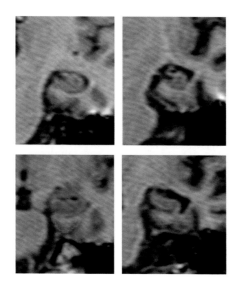

Fig. 1. MRI coronal section at the level of the hippocampus and EC. The location of the hippocampus within the brain is shown on the left. The images on the inside right show a normal hippocampus and EC (upper and lower images, respectively) compared to atrophic changes seen in AD (outside right).

SPECT determines cerebral perfusion by measuring the decay of a radioactive isotope. In AD, there is a pattern of decreased perfusion in the parietotemporal cortex, the hippocampus, the cingulate gyrus, and the thalamus with a sensitivity of 86% and a specificity of 80% when comparing AD to controls. Despite being more widely available and cheaper than PET, SPECT is limited by poor spatial resolution and lower accuracy in differentiating between dementias.

In functional MRI (fMRI), measurement of a blood oxygen level-dependent MR signal is used as an indirect measure of neuronal activity. While fMRI has great potential for elucidating changes in brain function in AD and other disease states at present fMRI remains a research tool and is not employed in clinical practice as a diagnostic tool. Task-free, or resting state, fMRI permits assessment of brain functional connectivity in the absence of any engagement in specific cognitive tasks to cause brain activation. This approach has identified several large-scale functional brain networks, and within these there is particular interest in the default mode network, which represents a functionally connected network that includes the MTL, precuneus, posterior cingulate gyrus, and lateral parietal, lateral temporal, and medial prefrontal regions. Task-free fMRI studies in AD have identified decreased functional connectivity within the posterior default mode network [25] accompanied by increased connectivity within the anterior default mode network, and may be observed in the presymptomatic and prodromal stages of disease. Task-specific fMRI measures patterns of activation while the subject performs a task in the scanner. Studies using memory tasks have shown that hippocampal and MTL temporal activation decreases with advancing AD, with the accompanying increase in prefrontal activity possibly representative of a compensatory mechanism. Longitudinal studies have also revealed that early hippocampal hyperactivation is a predictor of cognitive decline in patients with MCI and early AD [26].

Histological Imaging

Ligand PET imaging with 'Pittsburgh Compound B' (^{11}C-PiB) allows the in vivo visualization of extracellular amyloid pathology [27]. In early AD, amyloid deposition as seen using PiB is noted in the frontoparietal-temporal association cortices, overlapping both with the regions that subsequently become hypometabolic on FDG-PET and consistent with the distribution of extracellular amyloid as noted in pathological studies. Studies in earlier stages of AD have shown that amyloid deposition is present during the presymptomatic [16] and prodromal stages of disease. Longitudinal studies [28] have shown that positive PiB-PET scanning is predictive of conversion from MCI to AD and can also predict future onset of dementia in cognitively normal individuals. The diagnostic sensitivity of PiB-PET remains uncertain since it may also detect amyloid in vivo in patients with dementia with Lewy bodies, amyloid angiopathy (without cortical Alzheimer pathology), and senile plaques seen in normal ageing.

Widespread use of PiB is limited by its short half-life of only 20 min, and as such a number of ^{18}F-based ligands are being explored in view of the longer half-life of ^{18}F-based compounds. Studies to date have shown a good correlation between PiB and ^{18}F distribution in vivo [29]. In 2013 the US Alzheimer's Association issued guidelines that recommended amyloid imaging in one of three circumstances: persistent MCI when AD remained a possible diagnosis, atypical AD syndrome, and young-onset dementia [29].

Multimodal Brain Imaging

Each imaging modality provides different insights into the neurodegenerative changes that occur throughout the course of AD. As such, a combination of approaches using multimodal imaging may represent an optimal means of interrogating histological, structural, and functional indices of pathology (fig. 2) with superior diagnostic sensitivity and specificity for diagnosis.

Non-Alzheimer's Dementia

There are a number of non-AD neurodegenerative disorders causing dementia, in which the hippocampus is variably affected. Each is described in brief below.

Vascular Dementia

Vascular dementia is not a single disease, but a syndrome of cognitive change that results from accumulation of small- or large-vessel ischemic insults. There is a shared risk profile for cerebrovascular disease and AD, and these pathologies often coexist

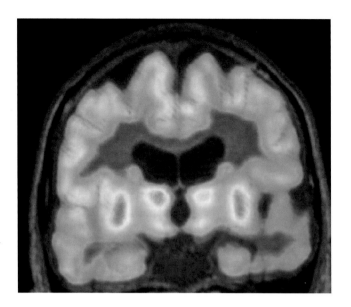

Fig. 2. Coregistered PET/MRI acquired simultaneously on an integrated PET-MRI scanner. This coronal section shows changes in a 75-year-old individual with mild AD. There is hippocampal atrophy accompanied by mild generalized cerebral atrophy. In addition to the MTL, there is extensive hypometabolism in the lateral temporal and dorsolateral frontal cortices.

especially in the elderly. In terms of clinical presentation, small vessel vascular dementia can mimic that of neurodegenerative disease, with progressive cognitive decline characterized by bradyphrenia, lower limb rigidity, and psychomotor slowing. Cerebrovascular insufficiency is known to accelerate the course of AD and also predisposes to hippocampal sclerosis, perhaps reflecting the vulnerability of CA1 to ischemia/hypoxia. Hippocampal atrophy may sometimes occur in vascular dementia, but is usually less severe than that seen in AD.

Dementia with Lewy Bodies

Dementia with Lewy bodies [30] is the second commonest cause of dementia after AD, and is characterized clinically by fluctuating cognitive impairment, visual hallucinations, and Parkinsonism. Histologically, there is accumulation of neuronal cytoplasmic inclusions (Lewy bodies) in the cerebral cortex, brainstem nuclei, and basal forebrain. The majority of cases also demonstrate the presence of extracellular Aβ deposition, but in the absence of NFTs. However, patients with dementia with Lewy bodies tend to be more impaired on tasks of verbal working memory and less impaired in terms of episodic verbal memory and working spatial memory than patients with AD. The degree of hippocampal atrophy found in dementia with Lewy bodies is less extensive than seen at a similar stage of AD.

Frontotemporal Lobar Degeneration

Frontotemporal lobar degeneration refers to a genetically, clinically, and pathologically diverse group of conditions that present with alterations in behavior, social conduct, executive function, speech, and language. Frontotemporal lobar degeneration is typically associated with a younger age of onset than AD. The anterior hippocampus is particularly affected in two of the clinical variants of frontotemporal lobar degeneration, namely the behavioral variant of frontotemporal dementia, in which there is apathy, dysexecutive functioning, and alterations in social comportment, and semantic dementia, which is characterized by impaired word meaning, anomia, and paraphasia with preserved episodic memory.

Dementia Syndromes in the Oldest Old

Argyrophilic grain disease, 'tangle-only' dementia, and hippocampal sclerosis are rare causes of cognitive decline, occurring more frequently in the elderly with an onset of symptoms beyond the age of 80 years. A common characteristic of these conditions is the shared expression of hyperphosphorylated tau inclusions in CA1 and the EC without the coexpression of dense amyloid pathology. Clinically, these may present with progressive impairment of episodic memory, but without the associated development of apraxia and aphasia typically seen in AD dementia. In argyrophilic grain disease there is additional involvement of the amygdala and the emergence of 'late-onset' schizophreniform symptoms, in excess of the delusional symptoms seen in AD. Tangle-only dementia shares the same pathology and topology of NFTs seen in Braak stage 4, but with less synaptic and neuronal loss, while hippocampal sclerosis may be acquired secondary to chronic epilepsy, head trauma, or vascular insufficiency.

Conclusion

Hippocampal involvement from the early stages of AD is central to the memory impairment that characterizes this disorder. In addition, the hippocampus is variably affected in non-AD dementias. Knowledge of this hippocampal involvement informs the design and application of diagnostic strategies with the aim of improving both diagnostic differentiation and identification of disease at earlier stages.

References

1 Schott JM, Fox NC, Frost C, Scahill RI, Janssen JC, Chan D, Jenkins RR, Rossor MN: Assessing the onset of structural change in familial Alzheimer's disease. Ann Neurol 2003;53:181–188.

2 Cataldo AM, Petanceska S, Terio NB, Peterhoff CM, Durham R, Mercken M, Mehta PD, Buxbaum J, Haroutunian V, Nixon RA: Abeta localization in abnormal endosomes: association with earliest Abeta elevations in AD and Down syndrome. Neurobiol Aging 2004;25:1263–1272.

3 Lesné SE, Sherman MA, Grant M, Kuskowski M, Schneider JA, Bennett DA, Ashe KH: Brain amyloid-β oligomers in ageing and Alzheimer's disease. Brain 2013;136:1383–1398.

4 Thal DR, Rüb U, Orantes M, Braak H: Phases of A beta-deposition in the human brain and its relevance for the development of AD. Neurology 2002;58:1791–1800.

5 Cacucci F, Yi M, Wills TJ, Chapman P, O'Keefe J: Place cell firing correlates with memory deficits and amyloid plaque burden in Tg2576 Alzheimer mouse model. Proc Natl Acad Sci USA 2008;105:7863–7868.

6 Hyman BT, Van Hoesen GW, Kromer LJ, Damasio AR: Perforant pathway changes and the memory impairment of Alzheimer's disease. Ann Neurol 1986; 20:472–481.

7 Liu L, Drouet V, Wu JW, Witter MP, Small SA, Clelland C, Duff K: Trans-synaptic spread of tau pathology in vivo. PLoS One 2012;7:e31302.

8 Braak H, Braak E: Neuropathological stageing of Alzheimer-related changes. Acta Neuropathol 1991;82: 239–259.

9 Giannakopoulos P, Herrmann FR, Bussiere T, Bouras C, Kovari E, Perl DP, Morrison JH, Gold G, Hof PR: Tangle and neuron numbers, but not amyloid load, predict cognitive status in Alzheimer's disease. Neurology 2003;60:1495–1500.

10 Tanzi RE, Bertram L: New frontiers in Alzheimer's disease genetics. Neuron 2001;32:181–184.

11 Hardy JA, Higgins GA: Alzheimer's disease: the amyloid cascade hypothesis. Science 1992;256:184–185.

12 Jonsson T, Atwal JK, Steinberg S, Snaedal J, Jonsson PV, Bjornsson S, Stefansson H, Sulem P, Gudbjartsson D, Maloney J, Hoyte K, Gustafson A, Liu Y, Lu Y, Bhangale T, Graham R, Huttenlocher J, Bjornsdottir G, Andreassen OA, Jönsson EG, Palotie A, Behrens TW, Magnusson OT, Kong A, Thorsteinsdottir U, Watts RJ, Stefansson K: A mutation in APP protects against Alzheimer's disease and age-related cognitive decline. Nature 2012;488:96–99.

13 Albert MS, DeKosky ST, Dickson D, Dubois B, Feldman HH, Fox NC, Gamst A, Holtzman DM, Jagust WJ, Petersen RC, Snyder PJ, Carrillo MC, Thies B, Phelps CH: The diagnosis of mild cognitive impairment due to Alzheimer's disease: recommendations from the National Institute on Aging-Alzheimer's Association workgroups on diagnostic guidelines for Alzheimer's disease. Alzheimers Dement 2011;7: 270–279.

14 McKhann GM, Knopman DS, Chertkow H, Hyman BT, Jack CR, Kawas CH, Klunk WE, Koroshetz WJ, Manly JJ, Mayeux R, Mohs RC, Morris JC, Rossor MN, Scheltens P, Carrillo MC, Thies B, Weintraub S, Phelps CH: The diagnosis of dementia due to Alzheimer's disease: recommendations from the National Institute on Aging-Alzheimer's Association workgroups on diagnostic guidelines for Alzheimer's disease. Alzheimers Dement 2011; 7:263–269.

15 Dubois B, Feldman HH, Jacova C, Cummings JL, DeKosky ST, Barberger-Gateau P, Delacourte A, Frisoni G, Fox NC, Galasko D, Gauthier S, Hampel H, Jicha GA, Meguro K, O'Brien J, Pasquier F, Robert P, Rossor M, Salloway S, Sarazin M, de Souza LC, Stern Y, Visser PJ, Scheltens P: Revising the definition of Alzheimer's disease: a new lexicon. Lancet Neurol 2010;9:1118–1127.

16 Bateman RJ, Xiong C, Benzinger TL, Fagan AM, Goate A, Fox NC, Marcus DS, Cairns NJ, Xie X, Blazey TM, Holtzman DM, Santacruz A, Buckles V, Oliver A, Moulder K, Aisen PS, Ghetti B, Klunk WE, McDade E, Martins RN, Masters CL, Mayeux R, Ringman JM, Rossor MN, Schofield PR, Sperling RA, Salloway S, Morris JC: Clinical and biomarker changes in dominantly inherited Alzheimer's disease. N Engl J Med 2012;367:795–804.

17 Pengas G, Patterson K, Arnold RJ, Bird CM, Burgess N, Nestor PJ: Lost and found: bespoke memory testing for Alzheimer's disease and semantic dementia. J Alzheimers Dis 2010;21:1347–1365.

18 Bird CM, Chan D, Hartley T, Pijnenburg YA, Rossor MN, Burgess N: Topographical short-term memory differentiates Alzheimer's disease from frontotemporal lobar degeneration. Hippocampus 2009;20: 1154–1169.

19 Folstein MF, Folstein SE, McHugh PR: 'Mini-mental state'. A practical method for grading the cognitive state of patients for the clinician. J Psychiatr Res 1975;12:189–198.

20 Mioshi E, Dawson K, Mitchell J, Arnold R, Hodges JR: The Addenbrooke's Cognitive Examination Revised (ACE-R): a brief cognitive test battery for dementia screening. Int J Geriatr Psychiatry 2006;21: 1078–1085.

21 Scheltens P, Fox N, Barkhof F, De Carli C: Structural magnetic resonance imaging in the practical assessment of dementia: beyond exclusion. Lancet Neurol 2002;1:13–21.

22 Jack CR, Petersen RC, Xu YC, Waring SC, O'Brien PC, Tangalos EG, Smith GE, Ivnik RJ, Kokmen E: Medial temporal atrophy on MRI in normal aging and very mild Alzheimer's disease. Neurology 1997; 49:786–794.

23 Chan D, Janssen JC, Whitwell JL, Watt HC, Jenkins R, Frost C, Rossor MN, Fox NC: Change in rates of cerebral atrophy over time in early-onset Alzheimer's disease: longitudinal MRI study. Lancet 2003; 362:1121–1122.

24 Mosconi L: Brain glucose metabolism in the early and specific diagnosis of Alzheimer's disease – FDG-PET studies in MCI and AD. Eur J Nucl Med Mol Imaging 2005;32:486–510.

25 Greicius MD, Srivastava G, Reiss AL, Menon V: Default-mode network activity distinguishes Alzheimer's disease from healthy aging: evidence from functional MRI. Proc Natl Acad Sci USA 2004;101: 4637–4642.
26 O'Brien JL, O'Keefe KM, LaViolette PS, DeLuca AN, Blacker D, Dickerson BC, Sperling RA: Longitudinal fMRI in elderly reveals loss of hippocampal activation with clinical decline. Neurology 2010;74:1969–1976.
27 Klunk WE, Engler H, Nordberg A, Wang Y, Blomqvist G, Holt DP, Bergström M, Savitcheva I, Huang G-F, Estrada S, Ausén B, Debnath ML, Barletta J, Price JC, Sandell J, Lopresti BJ, Wall A, Koivisto P, Antoni G, Mathis CA, Långström B: Imaging brain amyloid in Alzheimer's disease with Pittsburgh Compound-B. Ann Neurol 2004;55:306–319.
28 Villemagne VL, Burnham S, Bourgeat P, Brown B, Ellis KA, Salvado O, Szoeke C, Macaulay SL, Martins R, Maruff P, Ames D, Rowe CC, Masters CL, Australian Imaging Biomarkers and Lifestyle (AIBL) Research Group: Amyloid β deposition, neurodegeneration, and cognitive decline in sporadic Alzheimer's disease: a prospective cohort study. Lancet Neurol 2013;12:357–367.
29 Johnson KA, Minoshima S, Bohnen NI, Donohoe KJ, Foster NL, Herscovitch P, Karlawish JH, Rowe CC, Carrillo MC, Hartley DM, Hedrick S, Pappas V, Thies WH: Appropriate use criteria for amyloid PET: a report of the Amyloid Imaging Task Force, the Society of Nuclear Medicine and Molecular Imaging, and the Alzheimer's Association. Alzheimers Dement 2013;9:e1–e16.
30 McKeith IG: Consensus guidelines for the clinical and pathologic diagnosis of dementia with Lewy bodies (DLB): report of the Consortium on DLB International Workshop. J Alzheimers Dis 2006;9: 417–423.

Dr. Dennis Chan
Herchel Smith Building for Brain and Mind Sciences
University of Cambridge
Forvie Site, Robinson Way
Cambridge CB2 0SZ (UK)
E-Mail dc598@medschl.cam.ac.uk

Szabo K, Hennerici MG (eds): The Hippocampus in Clinical Neuroscience.
Front Neurol Neurosci. Basel, Karger, 2014, vol 34, pp 109–120 (DOI: 10.1159/000356423)

Stress, Memory, and the Hippocampus

Katja Wingenfeld[a] · Oliver T. Wolf[b]

[a]Department of Psychiatry, Charité University Berlin, Campus Benjamin Franklin, Berlin, and
[b]Cognitive Psychology, Institute of Cognitive Neuroscience, Ruhr University Bochum, Bochum,
Germany

Abstract

Stress hormones, i.e. cortisol in human and cortisone in rodents, influence a wide range of cognitive functions, including hippocampus-based declarative memory performance. Cortisol enhances memory consolidation, but impairs memory retrieval. In this context glucocorticoid receptor sensitivity and hippocampal integrity play an important role. This review integrates findings on the relationships between the hypothalamus-pituitary-adrenal (HPA) axis, one of the main coordinators of the stress response, hippocampus, and memory. Findings obtained in healthy participants will be compared with selected mental disorders, including major depressive disorder (MDD), posttraumatic stress disorder (PTSD), and borderline personality disorder (BPD). These disorders are characterized by alterations of the HPA axis and hippocampal dysfunctions. Interestingly, the acute effects of stress hormones on memory in psychiatric patients are different from those found in healthy humans. While cortisol administration has failed to affect memory retrieval in patients with MDD, patients with PTSD and BPD have been found to show enhanced rather than impaired memory retrieval after hydrocortisone. This indicates an altered sensitivity to stress hormones in these mental disorders.

Hypothalamus-Pituitary-Adrenal Axis

Stress, including traumatic experiences, is associated with dramatic increases in the risk of developing psychiatric and somatic disorders. Following the biopsychosocial model of mental disorders, many studies have focused on the functioning of the hypothalamic-pituitary-adrenal (HPA) axis, which is an important part of the neuroendocrine system involved in the coordination of the stress response. Briefly, upon stress exposure, corticotropin-releasing factor (CRF) is released from the hypothalamus and is transported to the anterior pituitary. There it stimulates the secretion of adrenocorticotropin (ACTH), which in turn stimulates the synthesis and release of glucocorticoids (GCs) from the adrenal cortex. The HPA axis is counterregulated by circulating GCs via negative feedback mechanisms targeting the pituitary, hypothalamus, hippocampus, and parts of the prefrontal cortex. The hippocampus exerts negative feedback on the paraventricular nucleus of the hypothalamus, thereby reducing HPA axis activity. This negative feedback loop is essential for the regulation of the HPA axis [1]. GCs mediate their effects by binding to two subtypes of intracellular receptors: the mineralocorticoid receptor (MR) and the glucocorticoid receptor (GR). These two receptors differ in their affinity and distribution within the brain: while the MR is mainly located in the hippocampus, the GR is not restricted to the hippocampus but expressed throughout the brain [1]. Recently, membrane-bound GRs and MRs have also been identified [2, 3]. Due to their prominence throughout the brain, corticoid receptors modulate several cognitive processes, including memory. While most of the effects associated with GCs – especially those that are related to stress – have been attributed to the GR, more recent studies have emphasized the importance of the MR [2].

Stress Hormones and Memory

In healthy participants, multiple investigations have found that acute administration of GCs impairs long-term memory retrieval. Similar effects have been obtained using psychosocial laboratory stressors. Memory consolidation, on the other hand, seems to be enhanced by cortisol [4].

Most studies on the effects of cortisol and stress on memory focus on behavioral measurement, i.e. memory performance, while only a few studies have investigated the neural correlates. Psychosocial stress has been reported to decrease activation in limbic areas including the hippocampus, hypothalamus, medial orbitofrontal cortex, and anterior cingulate cortex [5]. Furthermore, there is evidence for an increased activity in the amygdala and frontal brain areas in response to stress [5]. Intriguingly, hippocampus activation patterns in response to acute social stress are associated with the magnitude of the cortisol stress response: healthy participants who deactivated their hippocampal structure under stress responded to an acute social stressor with a stronger release of cortisol [5]. This observation is in line with the idea that the hippocampus has a tonic inhibitory impact on the HPA axis.

Some studies have applied pharmacological challenges (e.g. cortisol administration) in healthy participants during functional MRI to try to mimic the physiological stress response. Most of these studies found that exogenous administration of hydrocortisone leads to reduced activity in the hippocampus and prefrontal regions (e.g. [6], see fig. 1). However, it appears to be crucial to consider the time frame of the ef-

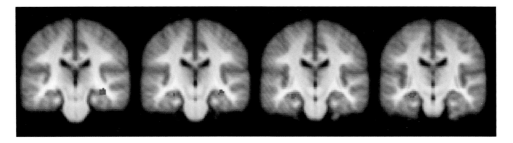

Fig. 1. Coronal slices showing the effects of cortisol on hippocampal activity during memory retrieval. Cortisol reduced activation as compared to placebo in the left and right hippocampus. Reprinted from Oei et al. [6] with permission of Springer Science and Business Media.

fects of cortisol when appraising these results. Cortisol leads to fast but short-lived increased excitability of the hippocampus before the inhibitory effects kick in [7]. In one functional MRI study, the slow effects of cortisol were shown to lead to reduced activity in the hippocampus and prefrontal cortex [8]. Another imaging study in healthy humans tested memory after a psychosocial stressor and found a stronger activation of the right anterior hippocampus during encoding, but a reduced activity in the left posterior hippocampus during memory retrieval [9]. In sum, behavioral and imaging studies support the notion that GCs exert opposing effects on memory consolidation and memory retrieval.

A recent study focused on the interplay between the hippocampus-dependent declarative memory system and the striatum-dependent procedural memory system by using a probabilistic classification learning task in which both systems were involved [10]. Acute stress resulted in a shift from hippocampal activity to striatal activity during successful task solving. This shift, which has also been observed using other learning and memory paradigms might be adaptive since it typically rescues performance. However, the acquired behavior is less flexible and more rigid [10]. In sum, GCs have profound effects on the quality and quantity of human memories. One important mechanism is the modulating effects of the stress hormone cortisol on hippocampal function.

Stress Hormones, Memory, and Psychiatric Disorders

Major Depressive Disorder

Major depressive disorder (MDD) is one of the most prevalent mental disorders. The main symptom of MDD is depressed mood and/or loss of interest or pleasure. Cognitive problems, including memory disturbances, are also frequent in patients with MDD. Hippocampal-based episodic/declarative memory as assessed by tasks like paragraph delayed recall and learning and retrieval of word lists is impaired in MDD patients [11]. Biological, psychological, and social factors are known to play a role in the development of MDD, suggesting that depression results when a preexisting vulnerability is activated by stressful life events [12].

Hypothalamic-Pituitary-Adrenal Axis Alterations in Major Depressive Disorder

In MDD, dysregulations of the HPA axis have been reported repeatedly. The most prominent findings have been enhanced basal and stimulated cortisol release and high cortisol concentrations after dexamethasone (DEX) administration, i.e. DEX nonsuppression, which indicates impaired negative feedback of the HPA axis [13]. This finding has been interpreted as reflecting an exaggerated CRF drive and/or as a reduction of functioning of GRs. One of the most sensitive measurements of HPA axis feedback sensitivity is the combined DEX/CRF test. In this test, HPA axis activity is initially suppressed by DEX treatment before exogenous CRF is given the following day. In depressed patients a pronounced escape from this suppression has been found with elevated ACTH and cortisol after CRF administration, supporting the idea of reduced GR functioning in these patients [14].

In line with the above-mentioned hypothesis that preexisting physiological risk factors in concert with psychosocial stressors contribute to the development of MDD [12], studies on gene-environment interactions are of interest. One way environmental factors, such as early life stress, may influence HPA axis regulation in later life is by altering the activity of genes via epigenetic mechanisms (e.g. methylation). In fact, postmortem studies in humans have not only reported reduced GR mRNA in depressed patients, but also increased methylation of the GR gene promoter inhibiting GR expression [15]. Furthermore, GR gene polymorphisms have been thought to be associated with depression. Traditionally, the GR has been at the focus of most studies examining neuroendocrine pathways to depression. However, recent evidence suggests that MR dysfunction might also play a role [1]. Future studies need to investigate the MR/GR imbalance model of depression using a combined investigations of both receptors.

Neuroimaging Findings in Major Depressive Disorder

Due to the high density of GR in the hippocampus, this brain structure is thought to be a brain region sensitive for the damaging effects of chronic stress or chronically elevated GCs [4]. In MDD, hippocampal volume reduction is a prominent finding, but several factors such as childhood trauma and illness duration seem to be associated with smaller hippocampal size [12]. Furthermore, when using functional imaging, deficits in hippocampal activation in patients with MDD in a verbal memory encoding task could be revealed [16]. To our knowledge, up to now there has been no functional imaging study that has investigated what happens at the neural level, especially the hippocampus, in response to a stressor or cortisol administration in MDD patients. In sum, findings of the research which investigate the hippocampus in MDD fit well to the hypothesis of an overactive HPA axis in these

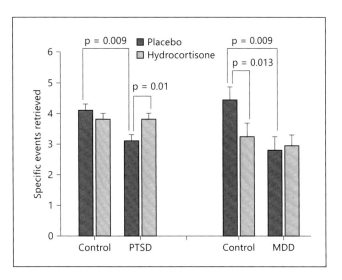

Fig. 2. Effects of 10 mg of hydrocortisone on autobiographical memory retrieval [autobiographic memory test, number of specific events retrieved; mean (SE)] in patients with PTSD and MDD in comparison to sex- and age-matched healthy controls. Adapted from Wingenfeld et al. [24] and Schlosser et al. [18] with permission from Elsevier.

patients. Both high cortisol concentrations in concert with reduced feedback sensitivity of the axis and hippocampal dysfunction might contribute to memory deficits in these patients.

Cortisol and Memory in Major Depressive Disorder

Several studies have investigated the association between HPA axis functioning and memory performance in depression. Some studies found associations between cortisol concentrations and cognitive impairment in depressed patients, while other studies failed to find such associations [17]. However, the cross-sectional and correlational designs of these studies preclude causal interpretations.

To our knowledge, only few studies have investigated the effect of acute GC administration on memory in MDD. We recently investigated the effect of a single administration of 10 mg of hydrocortisone on autobiographic memory retrieval in patients with MDD. These patients often show an overgeneralized memory style, i.e. they have difficulties retrieving specific autobiographical events; they tend to reply with abstract or general memory content (e.g. they summarize several different events). We found, in line with previous work, memory retrieval impairment in healthy controls after cortisol intake [18]. In patients with MDD, no such impairment was observed, but the two groups differed under placebo with MDD patients exhibiting worse memory (fig. 2). A similar pattern was seen in another declarative memory task, a word-list learning paradigm: while cortisol impaired memory retrieval in healthy participants, there was no effect seen in patients with MDD [19]. We hypothesized that the lack of an effect of acute cortisol administration on memory retrieval in MDD might be caused by reduced functioning (reduced sensitivity) of hippocampal and/or prefrontal GRs.

Taken together, MDD is characterized by HPA axis alterations, hippocampal volume reductions, and memory deficits. Moreover, there is a lack of effects of GCs on memory retrieval. How exactly these alterations are associated with each other remains to be determined. The finding of a reduced hippocampal volume might be a preexisting risk factor or a consequence of elevated cortisol exposure, and both might be associated with memory disturbances. Moreover, there is compelling evidence for GR dysfunction. Again, this might be a risk factor for the development of depression, possibly due to epigenetic factors in the context of early life adversities or a consequence of prolonged excessive cortisol release [12]. Future studies should integrate endocrine and cognitive methods with neuroimaging to investigate what happens in MDD patients on a neural level when exposed to acute stress or GCs. Furthermore, longitudinal studies are needed to disentangle risk factors and alterations due to the depressive state of the patients.

Posttraumatic Stress Disorder

Posttraumatic stress disorder (PTSD) follows exposure to a traumatic event, defined as a threat to one's life or someone close, associated with intense fear, horror, or helplessness. Traumatic experiences include childhood abuse, accidents, rape, assault, war, and natural disasters. PTSD is characterized by three distinct but cooccurring symptoms: reexperiencing the trauma, avoidance, and hyperarousal. Stress-induced changes in neurobiological systems (e.g. enhanced sensitization to stress and physiological hyperarousal) have been thought to contribute to PTSD symptoms and to disturbances in learning and memory in these patients. Of note, autobiographical memory is implicated in PTSD (e.g. in terms of intrusive memories) and neuropsychological alterations are an important feature of the clinical presentation of PTSD. Several studies have revealed learning and memory deficits, including impairments in declarative memory functions as well as reduced autobiographical memory specificity and overgeneralized memory [20].

Hypothalamic-Pituitary-Adrenal Axis Alterations in Posttraumatic Stress Disorder

As PTSD is clearly defined as a stress-related disorder, many studies have investigated the regulation of the HPA axis in PTSD. In contrast to MDD, cortisol findings in PTSD suggest reduced rather than enhanced basal concentrations [21]. However, these results are not consistent across all studies, and several factors, such as differences in trauma type, symptom patterns, gender, comorbidity with other mental disorders, and genetic and other predisposing factors have been thought to contribute to this inconsistency. Beyond so-called hypocortisolism, an enhanced suppression after a low dose (0.5 mg) of DEX has been reported repeatedly. This has been interpreted in the context of increased negative feedback regulation of the HPA axis due to increased GR binding [21]. At higher levels of the HPA axis, namely at the central nervous system, an increased concentration of CRF has been found [22]. The finding of a blunted ACTH response to exogenous CRF, possibly due to downregulation of pituitary CRF receptors, further supports the hypothesis of an enhanced activity of hypothalamic CRF [22]. Thus, the proposed CRF overdrive in PTSD in concert with altered function of the GR is under discussion in PTSD.

Neuroimaging Findings in Posttraumatic Stress Disorder

Several studies have reported reduced hippocampal size in PTSD patients [23]. This was formerly interpreted as a result of enhanced cortisol release in response to the trauma, but might also be a preexistent risk factor. Of note, adversities early in life may also contribute to hippocampal dysregulations and, thus, enhance the likelihood of developing PTSD in response to a trauma in adulthood. Furthermore, the cited meta-analyses reported that the structural brain abnormalities found in PTSD were moderated by MRI methodology, symptom severity, medication, age, and gender [23]. Thus, the cause of hippocampal abnormalities in PTSD needs further investigation.

Cortisol and Memory in Posttraumatic Stress Disorder

Studies that have investigated the effects of GC treatment on learning and memory in PTSD have yielded inconclusive results. One study reported a stronger negative effect of hydrocortisone on declarative memory in PTSD compared to controls. In older PTSD patients, further evidence for a more pronounced effect of cortisol was obtained, but this time enhanced working memory after hydrocortisone injection was observed. Another study reported that hydrocortisone led to an impaired hippocampal-dependent trace eyeblink conditioning in PTSD patients, but not in healthy control participants (reviewed in [20]).

In one of our own studies, we compared PTSD patients and healthy controls with respect to the effects of hydrocortisone on declarative memory retrieval by using an autobiographic memory test and word-list task. In both tests, opposing effects of cortisol on memory were observed when comparing patients with controls [24]. Cortisol had, as expected, impairing effects on memory retrieval in the controls, but enhancing effects on retrieval occurred in PTSD patients (fig. 2). These results suggest beneficial effects of cortisol on hippocampal-mediated memory processes in PTSD. This interpretation is supported by a neuroimaging study with veterans with PTSD. Here, administration of hydrocortisone resulted in enhanced activity of the hippocampus, which was not detected in control veterans without PTSD [25].

The finding of enhanced memory after cortisol treatment in PTSD patients shares similarities with recent observations in rodents. Rats which were exposed to stress early in life displayed impaired neuronal plasticity in adulthood. Interestingly, corticosterone treatment enhanced neuronal plasticity in the hippocampus (as assessed by long-term potentiation) in these animals, but impaired it in the control animals which did not have early life stress [26]. Thus, early adversity might influence the response of the hippocampus to GCs in adulthood, most likely via epigenetic mechanisms. As mentioned before, the effects of GCs on memory are mostly discussed in the context of GR functioning. The role of GR function in PTSD is still a matter of debate, but there is evidence that early trauma (i.e. history of sexual abuse) may induce epigenetic changes in hippocampal neurons affecting the GR via methylation of the GR gene [15]. However, this would suggest decreased GR sensitivity in PTSD. Interestingly, there is some evidence that cortisol treatment may reduce involuntary retrieval of traumatic memory, i.e. flashbacks [27]. Furthermore, beneficial effects of cortisol have been shown in the context of prevention of PTSD symptoms after acute trauma experiences [28]. As one can see, there is growing evidence for (in part) beneficial effects of cortisol in PTSD.

Borderline Personality Disorder: Psychopathology and Clinical Features

Borderline personality disorder (BPD) is characterized by intense and rapidly changing mood states as well as by impulsivity, self-injurious behaviors, fear of abandonment, unstable relationships, and unstable self-image. Patients with BPD frequently report early, multiple, and chronic adverse or traumatic experiences, such as repeated sexual or physical abuse or emotional or physical neglect. It has been suggested that early life stress might be an important risk factor in the development of BPD. Thus, alterations in the regulation of the HPA axis are of particular interest. Efforts to characterize neuropsychological functioning of BPD patients have yielded inconclusive results: while many studies have suggested significant impairment concerning episodic memory functioning, other studies have been unable to detect such deficits [20]. Interestingly, the pattern of results change when emotional valence is also considered in more sophisticated experimental designs, showing clearer deficits with higher task demands and/or emotional stress.

Hypothalamic-Pituitary-Adrenal Axis Alterations in Borderline Personality Disorder

Most studies investigating the HPA axis in BPD have focused on the feedback regulation of the axis by using the 1-mg DEX suppression test, which is comparable to research in MDD. The majority of these studies reported higher cortisol concentrations after DEX in BPD compared to healthy controls, but also suggested an association of reduced feedback inhibition with affective dysregulations or even with comorbid MDD [29]. In many studies, no clinical interview was performed to account for comorbid diagnosis, making the data difficult to interpret. More recent studies have used more appropriate diagnostic procedures as well as the low-dose (0.5 mg) DEX suppression test to also detect hypersuppression to DEX treatment as proposed for PTSD [21]. Again, the results remain heterogeneous with enhanced and reduced negative feedback regulation, but there is also evidence that comorbid disorders, such as MDD and PTSD, play an important role in terms of HPA feedback regulation in BPD [29]. Compared to other psychiatric disorders like MDD or PTSD, relatively few studies have investigated basal cortisol release, but the existing ones suggest enhanced cortisol concentrations [29]. Furthermore, an exaggerated ACTH and cortisol response in the combined DEX/CRF test has been found, but only among those who reported childhood abuse [30]. Again comorbid disorders, especially PTSD, seem to have an important influence on endocrine reactions [29].

To conclude, studies investigating how the HPA axis functions in BPD have provided evidence for the impact of comorbid PTSD and depression on HPA axis feedback regulation in BPD. One might hypothesize that BPD is not a simple diagnostic entity. It is possible that there are at least two subgroups of BPD patients with different endocrine patterns: one predominantly characterized by trauma-associated symptoms unaltered to enhanced feedback sensitivity and normal-to-reduced cortisol release, and another subgroup with mood disturbances as core symptoms and HPA axis dysfunction in the form of enhanced cortisol release and reduced feedback sensitivity.

Neuroimaging Findings in Borderline Personality Disorder

Consistent with the notion that BPD can be construed as a stress- or trauma-related disorder, several studies have investigated brain structures that are involved in memory as well as emotion and stress regulation, such as the hippocampus and the amygdala. The most consistent result is hippocampal volume reduction, while some but not all studies have also found smaller amygdala volumes [29]. The results of hippocampal volume loss are in line with the idea that stress, and especially early life stress, may have exerted a damaging effect on the brain in these patients. However, it is still a matter of debate whether reduced hippocampal volume is a consequence of stress or is genetically determined. Furthermore, in this context there are impressive similarities among BPD, PTSD, and MDD patients who also display hippocampal volume reduction. One might suggest that disturbances in hippocampal integrity, possibly due to early adverse experiences, might be a nonspecific risk factor for the development of psychiatric disorders.

Cortisol and Memory in Borderline Personality Disorder

In a recent study by our group, we investigated the effects of hydrocortisone on memory retrieval in 72 patients with BPD and 40 healthy controls in a placebo-controlled crossover design. Similar to our results in PTSD patients, cortisol enhanced rather that impaired memory retrieval in BPD patients [31]. Patients with BPD alone as well as BPD patients with comorbid PTSD showed this effect. Additionally, we found that comorbid MDD influenced the cortisol effects. In the subgroup of BPD patients with comorbid depression but no PTSD, the effects of cortisol on memory were absent, suggesting that these patients differ from other BPD patients in terms of their sensitivity to GCs. In sum, our results suggest an enhanced reactivity to exogenous cortisol in these patients. Alternatively, hydrocortisone might reduce brain activity in regions which are hyperactive in BPD, such as temporal areas. Due to the fact that this study is the only one which investigated the effects of cortisol on memory in BPD, the results need replication.

For borderline patients, a dysfunctional frontolimbic network including the amygdala, prefrontal areas, and other limbic structures (i.e. the anterior cingulate cortex and hippocampus) has been proposed from imaging [29]. However, the effects of cortisol administration on brain activity in BPD have not been investigated yet, so there is a need for functional neuroimaging studies illustrating the neural correlates of the described behavioral effects of acute cortisol administration.

Conclusion

In healthy humans, stress and GCs affect learning and memory, with impairing effects on memory retrieval and enhancing effects on memory consolidation. Several mental disorders, including MDD, PTSD, and BPD are characterized by dysfunctions of the HPA axis, hippocampal volume reduction, and memory disturbances, which might be associated with each other. Only a few studies have investigated the effects of cortisol (or stress) in these disorders. We showed that in contrast to healthy controls, cortisol did not show an effect on memory retrieval in patients with major depression. This might be behavioral evidence for a reduced function of central GRs. Many studies in MDD patients support this hypothesis. PTSD and BPD were found to have a completely different pattern of cortisol effects on memory: both patient groups showed an enhanced rather than impaired memory retrieval after cortisol. The interpretation of these findings is more challenging. One might suggest beneficial effects of acute cortisol elevations on hippocampal-mediated memory processes, possibly due to an enhanced GR function. However, findings on GR sensitivity in PTSD are inconclusive and for BPD patients such studies are missing completely. Furthermore, the role of the MR as well as the MR/GR balance in this context is not understood. Alternatively, memory improvement after cortisol administration could be interpreted in the context of inhibition of central CRF release through cortisol administration.

There is still the question of how this research is to be transferred into treatment strategies. As mentioned above, in PTSD there is some evidence that GC administration might reduce the retrieval of aversive memories [32], but more research is needed to draw final conclusions about the effectiveness and underlying mechanisms.

In major depression, much effort is currently directed at the development of pharmacological agents that may normalize HPA axis activity, with CRF and GR antagonists of particularly great interest [33]. In addition to pharmacological approaches, there is also preliminary evidence that HPA axis dysfunction in MDD patients can be altered via psychotherapy [34]. This is of importance for patients who are known to respond less to pharmacotherapy, i.e. MDD patients with a history of early trauma [35]. Furthermore, the longitudinal course of cortisol effects on memory would be of interest. Are the found alterations only seen during illness, e.g. in the depressive episode, or do they disappear when the patients recover?

In sum, despite the well-known effects of stress and GCs on memory, only a few studies have integrated the investigation of the HPA axis and cognitive function in mental disorders. Furthermore, in healthy humans, neuroimaging studies have helped us to understand the neural correlates of these effects. More neuroimaging studies in psychiatric patients are needed to localize brain regions showing altered sensitivity to stress hormones in these disorders. Finally, it would be of interest to test the impact of therapeutic interventions on these markers of central GC sensitivity.

References

1 de Kloet ER, Joels M, Holsboer F: Stress and the brain: from adaptation to disease. Nat Rev Neurosci 2005;6:463–475.

2 Joels M, et al: The coming out of the brain mineralocorticoid receptor. Trends Neurosci 2008;31:1–7.

3 Roozendaal B, et al: Membrane-associated glucocorticoid activity is necessary for modulation of long-term memory via chromatin modification. J Neurosci 2010;30:5037–5046.

4 Wolf OT: Stress and memory in humans: twelve years of progress? Brain Res 2009;1293:142–154.

5 Dedovic K, D'Aguiar C, Pruessner JC: What stress does to your brain: a review of neuroimaging studies. Can J Psychiatry 2009;54:6–15.

6 Oei NY, et al: Glucocorticoids decrease hippocampal and prefrontal activation during declarative memory retrieval in young men. Brain Imaging Behav 2007;1:31–41.

7 Joels M, Fernandez G, Roozendaal B: Stress and emotional memory: a matter of timing. Trends Cogn Sci 2011;15:280–288.

8 Henckens MJ, et al: Dynamically changing effects of corticosteroids on human hippocampal and prefrontal processing. Hum Brain Mapp 2012;33:2885–2897.

9 Weerda R, et al: Effects of acute psychosocial stress on working memory related brain activity in men. Hum Brain Mapp 2010;31:1418–1429.

10 Schwabe L, Wolf OT: Stress and multiple memory systems: from 'thinking' to 'doing'. Trends Cogn Sci 2013;17:60–68.

11 Chamberlain SR, Sahakian BJ: The neuropsychology of mood disorders. Curr Psychiatry Rep 2006;8:458–463.

12 Heim C, Binder EB: Current research trends in early life stress and depression: review of human studies on sensitive periods, gene-environment interactions, and epigenetics. Exp Neurol 2012;233:102–111.

13 Parker KJ, Schatzberg AF, Lyons DM: Neuroendocrine aspects of hypercortisolism in major depression. Horm Behav 2003;43:60–66.

14 Ising M, et al: The combined dexamethasone/CRH test as a potential surrogate marker in depression. Prog Neuropsychopharmacol Biol Psychiatry 2005;29:1085–1093.

15 McGowan PO, et al: Epigenetic regulation of the glucocorticoid receptor in human brain associates with childhood abuse. Nat Neurosci 2009;12:342–348.

16 Bremner JD, et al: Deficits in hippocampal and anterior cingulate functioning during verbal declarative memory encoding in midlife major depression. Am J Psychiatry 2004;161:637–645.

17 Schlosser N, Wolf OT, Wingenfeld K: Cognitive correlates of HPA axis alterations and their relevance for therapeutic interventions in major depressive disorder. Expert Rev Endocrinol Metab 2011;6:109–126.

18 Schlosser N, et al: Effects of acute cortisol administration on autobiographical memory in patients with major depression and healthy controls. Psychoneuroendocrinology 2010;35:316–320.

19 Terfehr K, et al: Effects of acute hydrocortisone administration on declarative memory in patients with major depressive disorder: a placebo-controlled, double-blind crossover study. J Clin Psychiatry 2011;72:1644–1650.

20 Wingenfeld K, Wolf OT: HPA axis alterations in mental disorders: impact on memory and its relevance for therapeutic interventions. CNS Neurosci Ther 2011;17:714–722.

21 Yehuda R: Status of glucocorticoid alterations in post-traumatic stress disorder. Ann NY Acad Sci 2009;1179:56–69.

22 Heim C, Nemeroff CB: Neurobiology of posttraumatic stress disorder. CNS Spectr 2009;14(1 suppl):13–24.

23 Karl A, et al: A meta-analysis of structural brain abnormalities in PTSD. Neurosci Biobehav Rev 2006;30:1004–1031.

24 Wingenfeld K, et al: Cortisol has enhancing, rather than impairing effects on memory retrieval in PTSD. Psychoneuroendocrinology 2012;37:1048–1056.

25 Yehuda R, et al: Hydrocortisone responsiveness in Gulf War veterans with PTSD: effects on ACTH, declarative memory hippocampal [(18)F]FDG uptake on PET. Psychiatry Res 2010;184:117–127.

26 Champagne DL, et al: Maternal care and hippocampal plasticity: evidence for experience-dependent structural plasticity, altered synaptic functioning, and differential responsiveness to glucocorticoids and stress. J Neurosci 2008;28:6037–6045.

27 Aerni A, et al: Low-dose cortisol for symptoms of posttraumatic stress disorder. Am J Psychiatry 2004;161:1488–1490.

28 Schelling G, et al: Efficacy of hydrocortisone in preventing posttraumatic stress disorder following critical illness and major surgery. Ann NY Acad Sci 2006;1071:46–53.

29 Wingenfeld K, et al: Borderline personality disorder: hypothalamus pituitary adrenal axis and findings from neuroimaging studies. Psychoneuroendocrinology 2010;35:154–170.

30 Rinne T, et al: Hyperresponsiveness of hypothalamic-pituitary-adrenal axis to combined dexamethasone/corticotropin-releasing hormone challenge in female borderline personality disorder subjects with a history of sustained childhood abuse. Biol Psychiatry 2002;52:1102–1112.

31 Wingenfeld K, et al: Effects of cortisol on memory in women with borderline personality disorder: role of comorbid posttraumatic stress disorder and major depression. Psychol Med 2013;43:495–505.

32 de Quervain DJ, et al: Glucocorticoids and the regulation of memory in health and disease. Front Neuroendocrinol 2009;30:358–370.

33 Schüle C: Neuroendocrinological mechanisms of actions of antidepressant drugs. J Neuroendocrinol 2007;19:213–226.

34 Yang TT, et al: The effect of psychotherapy added to pharmacotherapy on cortisol responses in outpatients with major depressive disorder. J Nerv Ment Dis 2009;197:401–406.

35 Nemeroff CB, et al: Differential responses to psychotherapy versus pharmacotherapy in patients with chronic forms of major depression and childhood trauma. Proc Natl Acad Sci USA 2003;100:14293–14296.

Prof. Dr. Oliver T. Wolf
Department of Cognitive Psychology, Ruhr University Bochum, GAFO 02/386
Universitätsstrasse 150
DE–44780 Bochum (Germany)
E-Mail oliver.t.wolf@rub.de

Szabo K, Hennerici MG (eds): The Hippocampus in Clinical Neuroscience.
Front Neurol Neurosci. Basel, Karger, 2014, vol 34, pp 121–142 (DOI: 10.1159/000356435)

Epilepsy and the Hippocampus

Anastasios Chatzikonstantinou

Department of Neurology, UniversitätsMedizin Mannheim, University of Heidelberg, Mannheim, Germany

Abstract

The association between epilepsy and the hippocampus is well known and important. Mesial temporal epilepsy with hippocampal sclerosis is a syndromic diagnostic entity and indeed a quite common one. There are different theories on the pathophysiological pathways, as the hippocampus is often involved in seizures, even if they are not generated there. Whether hippocampal sclerosis is a cause or the effect of seizures is a subject of ongoing debate, but the predominant opinion is that seizures probably do not cause relevant hippocampal volume loss in the mature brain. A diagnosis of epilepsy with hippocampal sclerosis is made based on typical semiological signs and symptoms, interictal and ictal EEG findings, cerebral imaging, and neuropsychological testing. Antiepileptic medication is indicated as a first-line treatment. Should the epilepsy prove to be medically intractable, which is commonly the case in these patients, an early evaluation regarding epilepsy surgery must be performed. Different epilepsy surgery techniques are available, from minimal ones like the selective amygdalohippocampectomy to more extensive ones like additional temporal lobe resection. Postoperative results concerning seizures and neuropsychological outcomes are very encouraging and depend on various predictive factors. Alternative procedures like stereotactic radiofrequency amygdalohippocampectomy and hippocampal stimulation are currently being assessed, partly with very promising results.

© 2014 S. Karger AG, Basel

History

There is a strong association between epilepsy and the hippocampus. In fact, hippocampal sclerosis is the most common pathological finding (60–70% of cases) in mesial temporal lobe epilepsy (MTLE), which in turn represents about 60% of all epilepsies with focal seizures. MTLE with hippocampal sclerosis (MTLE-HS) is widely accepted as a syndromic diagnostic entity, as it represents a unique cluster of signs and symptoms [1]. MTLE is significantly associated with a higher incidence of complicated febrile seizures [2–4]. The majority of patients undergoing epilepsy surgery for intractable partial seizures have been shown to have hippocampal sclerosis, other pathologies like focal cortical dysplasias, glioneuronal tumors, and vascular or traumatic lesions are considerably more rare. This association has been known since the 19th century, when pathologists (notably Bouchet and Cazauvieilh, 1825) noted changes in the hippocampus in epilepsy patients and the hippocampal sclerosis was described in detail. A causal relationship with epilepsy was postulated by John H. Jackson in the 1880s; he also described the semiology of seizures in detail. This causal relationship was supported by the good surgical outcome of temporal lobectomies performed by Falconer in the 1950s. Studies from the 1960s investigating hippocampal electrical activity showed that seizure-like electrical activity patterns are a significant feature of the hippocampus. Furthermore, it is very easy to experimentally manipulate the hippocampus to produce ictal discharges.

However, it remains unclear whether hippocampal sclerosis is a cause or an effect of epilepsy. There is strong evidence that hippocampal changes cause seizures: experimental studies with limbic kindling and intrahippocampal injections have resulted in triggering seizures, hippocampal sclerosis is linked to certain seizure types, surface and intracranial EEG data from long-term video-EEG monitoring suggest seizure onset in the hippocampus in many patients, and hippocampal resection in selected patients with temporal lobe epilepsy has shown excellent results regarding postoperative seizure control. On the other hand, several animal models and MRI and histopathological studies in humans have demonstrated that hippocampal sclerosis can be acquired as an effect of seizures, most evidently in the case of status epilepticus.

Evidence suggests that seizure onset in MTLE-HS occurs earlier than for other types of MTLE. Most patients have an epilepsy onset between 4 and 16 years of age, although there is a great variety [1]. A so-called 'silent period' between the first seizure and the onset of intractability is known to exist in a high percentage of patients, which could mean that the disease is progressive [1, 5]. Progressive memory and behavioral disorders as well as increased frequency of interictal epileptiform discharges also support this notion [1].

Seizure Semiology

The constellation of seizure semiology and EEG is quite distinctive in MTLE-HS. The new classification of seizures and electroclinical syndromes, suggested recently by the International League against Epilepsy, takes this into consideration and lists this epilepsy as an individual syndrome [6].

The temporal lobe is the most frequent origin of focal seizures. Temporal lobe seizures can be 'simple focal' (without impaired consciousness), 'complex focal' (with impaired consciousness), or secondarily generalized. Secondarily generalized seizures are reported to be not very common in antiepileptically treated patients with MTLE-HS because the medication suppresses secondary generalization better than focal seizures [1]. Temporal lobe seizures may originate in the hippocampus or from extrahippocampal neocortical temporal regions. Discrimination between temporal epilepsy with or without hippocampal sclerosis depending on seizure semiology alone can be very challenging, as there are no specific semiological signs and symptoms that are definitely associated with hippocampal sclerosis [1]. Studies utilizing (invasive) video-EEG monitoring, brain imaging, and pathophysiological results have demonstrated that some seizure semiology characteristics are typical for mesial temporal epilepsy (with hippocampal involvement) rather than for extrahippocampal seizures [2].

Many patients with MTLE (up to about 80% in the literature [2]) experience auras, which are focal seizures without impairment of consciousness. They can be isolated or, most commonly, precede complex focal seizures. Epigastric auras, i.e. auras with a rising epigastric sensation, gustatory and olfactory auras, auras with complex visual and complex or elementary auditory hallucinations, and auras with experiential phenomena such as déjà vu or jamais vu, are described as relatively specific for temporal lobe epilepsy [2, 7–11]. Epigastric auras have been shown to have a significant association with a mesial temporal rather than neocortical seizure origin [2, 10]. Epigastric auras are the most common auras in MTLE-HS and are found in about 65–70% of patients with MTLE [1, 9], followed by nonspecific auras, fear and anxiety (about 15–50% of cases), déjà vu or jamais vu auras (about 20–30% of cases), autonomous-vegetative auras, olfactory or gustatory auras (<5%), and abdominal pain with fear (in children) [1]. Epigastric, gustatory, and olfactory auras have been shown to be significantly more frequent in patients with MTLE-HS than in those with other temporal epilepsies [12]. Thus, auras can have a localizing significance, even within the temporal lobe. However, a lateralizing significance is usually absent [7].

The complex focal seizure usually begins with motionless staring and behavioral arrest; consciousness and/or awareness are impaired, commonly for a period of up to 2 min. Impairment or alteration of consciousness is interindividually different and often difficult to quantify. Automatisms, which describe an involuntary stereotyped motor activity, are a very common feature. Oral automatisms, such as chewing or smacking, are common in the beginning of the seizure. These early automatisms correlate with a mesial temporal seizure onset, whereas early motor involvement of the contralateral upper extremity without oral automatisms is a hint against a hippocampal and for a neocortical seizure onset. Other automatisms, most often gestural (like fumbling or fidgeting with the hands) are also very common. Other motor features, such as dystonic posturing and cloni, can also occur. These features seem to be more common in extrahippocampal seizures. This is probably because, due to the strong inhibitory mechanisms of the dentate gyrus and the relatively restricted connectivity, ictal activity usually remains confined to the hippocampus; if a propagation takes place, then it is commonly to the basal ganglia, resulting in a contralateral dystonic posturing [10, 13–15]. Patients are amnestic for the duration of the complex partial seizure and often for some time postictally, whereas the aura is usually recalled.

Some of the semiological features have lateralizing value: head deviation at seizure onset is ipsilateral to the seizure focus, whereas it is contralateral when it occurs late in the seizure [2, 7, 16, 17]. Unilateral automatisms have been shown to be ipsilateral to the seizure focus (in mesial temporal epilepsy) and dystonic posturing contralateral to it. Postictal aphasia or dysphasia are signs of a seizure onset in the dominant hemisphere.

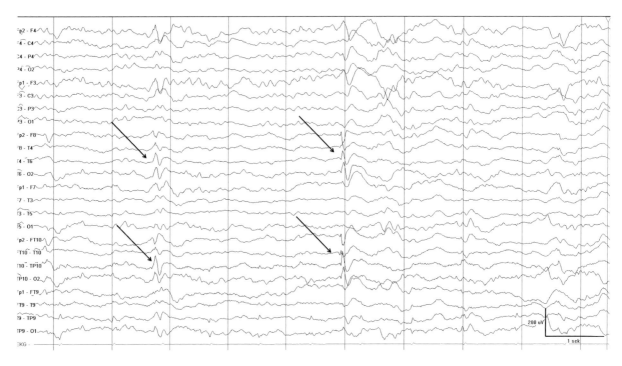

Fig. 1. Interictal EEG showing right temporal sharp waves.

Clinical Example

A 40-year-old, right-handed male patient presented himself in the outpatient department and reported having epilepsy since he was 23 years of age. He reported an olfactory aura and amnesia for the rest of the seizure. His wife described focal seizures with loss of consciousness, oral and manual (right hand) automatisms, and a frequency of about one seizure per week. Secondary generalizations were rare. The seizures were medically refractory, and antiepileptic medication included levetiracetam, lamotrigine, clobazam, and valproate. At the time of the first presentation, the patient was on high-dose levetiracetam (4,000 mg/day) and valproate (2,100 mg/day). Increased fatigue and aggressive tendencies were reported under this medication. No other disease was known and no other medication was taken. The patient was unemployed and had previously owned a grocery store, which he had to give up because of seizures and cognitive deficits. His family history was void of epilepsy.

During the video-EEG monitoring, an interictal focal theta-delta slowing with common sharp-slow waves was found in the right temporal region (F8, FT10, T4, T6, T10; fig. 1). Two habitual focal seizures with the described semiology could be recorded, showing a right temporal onset (F8, FT10, T4, T10) with rhythmic delta activity and a fast propagation to the right frontal and parietal lobes and, a few seconds later, to the contralateral hemisphere (fig. 2).

MRI showed significant volume loss of the right hippocampus with a hyperintense signal in the T2-weighted and MP-RAGE images (fig. 3). Additionally, in the 3-tesla images, parts of the adjacent temporal lobe also appeared slightly hyperintense, suggesting a possible additional lesion apart from the atrophic hippocampus. Neuropsychological examinations revealed deficits in verbal and visuospatial memory consolidation, as well as – to a lesser extent – impairment of semantic word fluency and selective attention.

Chatzikonstantinou

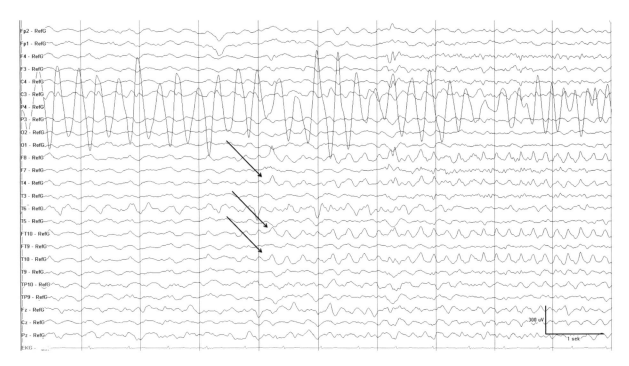

Fig. 2. Ictal EEG showing the seizure onset on the right temporal electrodes (movement artifact on electrode P4).

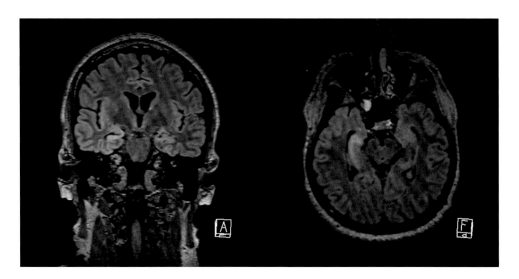

Fig. 3. Coronal and transversal MP-RAGE images showing volume loss and hyperintense signal of the right hippocampus.

The diagnosis of mesial temporal epilepsy with hippocampal sclerosis was made based on seizure semiology, EEG findings with interictal right temporal abnormalities and ictal onset on the right temporal lobe, neuropsychological deficits in accordance with hippocampal dysfunction, and – last but not least – the MRI findings of an altered right hippocampus.

After discussion of the case during an interdisciplinary epilepsy surgery meeting, a 2/3 temporal lobe resection with amygdalohippocampectomy was suggested. The additional temporal lobe resection was justified by the changes found by MRI involving part of the temporal lobe outside of the hippocampal region. Surgery was performed without complications. The patient has remained seizure free postoperatively, which at the time of writing has now been 1 year after the procedure. Valproate could be tapered off without problems, resulting in improved alertness of the patients. Levetiracetam is planned to be tapered carefully within the next months.

Etiology and Pathophysiology

Although the connection between hippocampal sclerosis and temporal lobe epilepsy is well known and undisputed, it remains unclear whether hippocampal sclerosis is a cause or an effect of epilepsy.

Initial Precipitating Incidents

There is indeed a high incidence of so-called 'initial precipitating incidents' in patients with MTLE-HS [18]. These include febrile seizures, hypoxia, head trauma, and meningitis/encephalitis in early age [1]. This is not unique to MTLE-HS, as patients with other types of MTLE also have in some cases a history of such incidents. Because of their high incidence, it was previously believed that these initial precipitating incidents, above all the febrile seizures, meant a higher risk for hippocampal sclerosis and epilepsy. However, studies have shown that the risk of epilepsy in children with febrile seizures is not significantly increased, although a causal relationship between atypical febrile seizures (such as focal seizures and/or long duration) and later epilepsy remains probable [19–22]. No prospective studies have proven the relation of any initial precipitating incidents to the later appearance of MTLE-HS and at least one third of the patients with hippocampal sclerosis have no known initial precipitating insult. An alternative hypothesis postulates that a preexisting temporal lobe abnormality that leads to hippocampal sclerosis later in life also increases the risk of febrile seizures in early age [23].

Pathogenesis of Hippocampal Sclerosis

There are a number of theories on the development of hippocampal sclerosis independently of epilepsy. Among others, glutamate neurotoxicity and mitochondrial dysfunction have been discussed [24], along with inflammatory and immunological factors [25], but the exact pathways of cell destruction remain unclear. Another hypothesis suggests that hippocampal sclerosis could be a developmental disorder based on the persistence of Cajal-Retzius cells and increased neurogenesis with an abnormal architectural organization of the dentate granule cell layer [26]. A genetic predisposition is also considered possible by a number of authors. Familial mesial temporal epilepsy has been described as a heterogeneous syndrome [27], and hippocampal abnormalities on MRI have been described in asymptomatic relatives of patients with MTLE-HS [28]. In animal models, sodium channel defects can cause hippocampal sclerosis; it is considered possible that such genetically defined defects could also play a role in the development of hippocampal sclerosis in humans.

Epileptogenesis in Hippocampal Sclerosis

There are currently two dominant theories about the epileptogenesis in the sclerotic hippocampus. The 'dormant basket cell' hypothesis suggests that inhibitory basket cells become 'dormant', i.e. hypofunctional due to loss of excitatory input from defect dentate mossy cells and other neurons in the same region. With the absence of their inhibitory (GABA-mediated) action, excitatory input can lead to excessive neuronal activity, neuronal death, and formation of an epileptic focus [29–31]. The 'mossy fiber' theory advocates that aberrant mossy fiber sprouting originating in the dentate granule cells and terminating in the supragranular region of the inner molecular layer of the fascia dentate causes electrophysiological dysfunction with formation of excitatory circuits resulting in hyperexcitability and spike generation [29, 32]. This mossy fiber sprouting has been detected in kainic acid epilepsy models in rats [33] and also in sclerotic hippocampi from human epilepsy surgery resections [34]. The actual and individual role of the numerous pathologic hippocampal changes that have been described in epileptogenesis cannot currently be determined and is the subject of ongoing research.

Hippocampal Sclerosis as a Result of Seizures?

Several animal studies have shown that hippocampal sclerosis can be caused by epileptic seizures, with the pathological features being similar to those in humans with MTLE-HS [29, 35]. Especially in kainic acid animal models, seizures provoked by kainic acid administration lead to hippocampal damage, which in turn produces unprovoked seizures [29, 36]. In the kindling model, repeated electrical stimulation of the hippocampus leads to neuronal loss in this area [37]. An increase of glutamate concentration in the sclerotic hippocampus during focal seizures has been described, which is theoretically capable of inducing neuronal damage [29]. MRI studies and postmortem examinations also indicate that status epilepticus can cause acute hippocampal dysfunction and damage [22, 38, 39]. Furthermore, progressive atrophy of the primarily affected and also the contralateral hippocampus in the course of MTLE has been shown [40, 41], although a correlation with the duration of epilepsy or the frequency and severity of seizures could not be prospectively confirmed [42].

However, most authors and experts nowadays agree that seizures do not necessarily damage the brain and that hippocampal sclerosis does not result from repeated seizures, at least in the mature brain [1, 43]. There is no good evidence that hippocampal sclerosis is progressive over time [44]. Few patients with newly diagnosed epilepsy (other than MTLE-HS) have visually detectable hippocampal atrophy [20]. Studies that have examined such patients over a period of years found very few cases of newly acquired hippocampal atrophy [20, 45, 46]. Volume declines, if detected, have been very modest [45].

Pathological Findings
The pathological changes of neuronal loss in the hippocampus in patients with epilepsy were first described in 1880 [29]. The International League against Epilepsy proposed in 2004 that the minimal criteria of MTLE-HS should be neuronal cell loss and gliosis at the CA1 and end-folium areas of the hippocampus with relative sparing of the transitional cortex measured at the mid-body of the anterior-posterior axis [1]. Further features include functional and structural glial changes, synaptic reorganization, dentate dispersion, and extrahippocampal changes, most commonly in the amygdala and the temporal white matter [1, 47, 48]. Moreover, there is data supporting the hypothesis that hippocampal sclerosis is often bilateral, but asymmetrical [18]. However, it remains unclear whether changes of the contralateral (less affected) hippocampus could be secondary, as a consequence of seizures. A simple classification of hippocampal sclerosis by Thom [23] includes the following subtypes and pathological features: (1) classical = neuronal loss and gliosis mainly in CA1, CA3, and end-folium, (2) total = severe neuronal loss in all hippocampal subfields and the dentate gyrus, and (3) end-folium = neuronal loss and gliosis restricted to the hilum of the dentate gyrus.

Diagnostic Work-Up

Seizure semiology plays an important role in differentiating focal seizures originating from the temporal lobe. Although the differentiation between an origin from the hippocampus in contrast to neocortical temporal areas is often difficult and can be based only on a handful of characteristics, as described above, (mesial) temporal lobe seizures can be distinguished quite well from seizures with onset in other parts of the brain. Seizures with early convulsive focal motor symptoms or with visual signs or associated with other neurological and neuropsychological deficits other than memory impairment are less likely to be of temporal origin. Thus, in patients with a suitable seizure pattern, a highly reliable diagnosis can be made utilizing EEG and MRI findings.

EEG
Video-EEG monitoring is usually performed to assess seizure semiology as well as ictal and interictal EEG. This modality is necessary for evaluation preceding a possible surgical treatment of epilepsy.

Scalp EEG recordings commonly show regional interictal slowing in about 50% of cases, which has a good lateralizing value [49, 50]. Also of high lateralizing value are interictal paroxysmal activity patterns [50]. Typical interictal epileptiform potentials in MTLE-HS are sharp waves or spikes with a field maximum in the temporal electrodes (T4/F8 or T3/F7). These include temporal spikes and are even better detected using sphenoidal electrodes, and can be confined unilaterally or spread to the contralateral temporal lobe. In many cases, these potentials are seen more often during drowsiness or sleep [1, 50]. Some findings suggest that the localization of interictal spikes can in some cases differentiate between mesial and neocortical temporal epilepsy [10]. The typical ictal EEG pattern consists of a rhythmic activity of 5–7/s at seizure onset or a few seconds later, in the temporal electrodes [51].

In most cases, the diagnosis of MTLE is done noninvasively. However, in patients in whom the lateralization or exact localization of the seizure focus is unclear, video-EEG monitoring with intracranial electrodes is used. EEG recorded with intracranial electrodes, which can also be placed inside the hippocampus, can confirm the localization of seizure focus and have revealed more details of ictal activity in the hippocampus. A usual ictal discharge pattern recorded using depth hippocampal electrodes is a low-amplitude, fast-activity discharge [52, 53]. The location of the onset of the ictal discharge in the hippocampus can vary within the same patient [52, 53]. Seizure propagation in MTLE-HS is thought to be relatively slow and to follow certain propagation pathways [1].

Imaging

MRI is essential in diagnosing possible hippocampal sclerosis. Its value in detecting hippocampal anomalies including sclerosis was acknowledged in the early 1990s [54, 55]. The usual findings are a unilateral hippocampal atrophy (in 90–95% of cases in which hippocampal sclerosis is found in resected tissue), accompanied by a hyperintense signal in FLAIR images on the pathological side (in 80–85% of cases). Additional typical hippocampal abnormalities are loss of internal architecture (in 60–95% of cases) and hypodensity in T1-weighted images [1, 56–58]. It has been demonstrated that reduced hippocampal volumes as measured on MRI indeed correlate with lower hippocampal neuronal cell quantities [59, 60]. Hippocampal volumes can be measured either manually [57] or automatically; however, manual measurements by an expert are considered to be superior to automated ones [61]. As FLAIR imaging enhances the hyperintense signal in hippocampal sclerosis (which is thought to represent gliosis) and can thus produce false-positive results, it is recommended that findings should additionally be confirmed using T2-weighted images [62]. T1-weighted images should be used to evaluate the anatomy and provide a good differentiation between white and gray matter. A hyperintense hippocampus in diffusion-weighted images indicates involvement of the hippocampus especially in prolonged seizures, as is discussed in the chapter by Szabo et al. [this vol., pp. 80–81].

Other features, such as temporal lobe atrophy and dilatation of the temporal horn, as well as atrophy of the fornix, mammillary body, insula, and thalamus may also be present [62, 63]. Additionally, epileptogenic lesions should also be looked for in any case. Associations with temporal lobe or hemispheric atrophy, low-grade tumors, ischemic lesions, and vascular or cortical malformations have been shown in the literature and are ipsilateral to the hippocampal sclerosis in most cases [64]. Another so-called case of 'dual pathology' is the presence of bilateral hippocampal sclerosis, which can represent a diagnostic challenge because of the possibly missing hippocampal asymmetry. Here, measurement of hippocampal volume can be particularly useful.

When evaluating the MRI, one should bear in mind that hippocampal asymmetry as well as hippocampal hyperintense signal in T2-weighted images can also be found in a normal population. According to the literature, a unilateral enlarged temporal horn occurs in about one third of healthy controls and should not be considered as a pathologic finding [65]. Either unilateral or bilateral hippocampal hyperintensities are encountered in about one third of normal controls, but without concomitant hippocampal atrophy [66].

For most cases, images from a standard 1.5-tesla scanner are sufficient [67]. However, high-resolution MRI (3 T) can be of great benefit when in search of a possible dual pathology, such as cortical dysplasias. The standard MRI protocol for epilepsy includes coronal images vertical to the hippocampal axis [62]. MRI protocols for epilepsy patients should be performed in a 1.5- or 3-tesla scanner with a slice thickness of 1.5–3 mm and should include 3D-T1 isotrope, T2* (hemosensitive), T2 axial, T2 coronar, FLAIR axial, and FLAIR coronar sequences. Standard MRI evaluated by nonexperts regarding epilepsy imaging can lead to false-negative results in up to about 60% of cases [62, 68].

MR spectroscopy detects peaks of concentrations of neuronal markers for neuronal loss, such as N-acetyl-aspartate, which is typically reduced in hippocampal sclerosis [69, 70]. The role and value of MR spectroscopy in the presurgical epilepsy evaluation of a patient with presumed hippocampal pathology is disputed, with conflicting data especially regarding MR-negative patients [71]. There is, however, evidence that a combination of MR spectroscopy and MR volumetry can help to lateralize temporal lobe epilepsy more securely [72].

Functional MRI (fMRI) is a method widely used to assess brain functions such as speech. Assessing the hippocampal functional reserve before a hippocampectomy could be very useful in predicting the risk of postsurgical neuropsychological deficits such as amnesia. However, current fMRI memory paradigms are not considered very reliable. New techniques like multivoxel pattern analysis could be more helpful in indicating hippocampal functional reserve [73].

PET, usually utilizing ^{18}F-fluorodeoxyglucose (FDG-PET), has played a role as an additional seizure focus-localizing imaging technique since the 1990s [74]. In mesial temporal epilepsy due to hippocampal sclerosis, the usual finding is regional interictal glucose hypometabolism of mesial temporal structures [75]. The pathophysiology behind this feature is not entirely understood [62, 76–78]. PET is widely used in presurgical epilepsy evaluation. A meta-analysis from 24 epilepsy centers showed that ipsilateral glucose hypometabolism had a predictive value of 86% for positive postsurgical outcome [79]. However, the additional advantage of PET is limited or negligible when hippocampal sclerosis can be identified as the seizure focus by video-EEG monitoring and MRI. Nevertheless, it can be helpful in cases with normal MRI [79]. In these MRI-negative patients, another ^{11}C-flumazenil-PET (FMZ-PET) can be also useful, although it is not widely used because of its high cost and the limited availability of the tracer. FMZ is a marker for $GABA_A$ and benzodiazepine receptors, and thus indirectly a marker for (hippocampal) neuronal cell loss [62]. It has been shown that FMZ-PET-positive patients without detection of hippocampal anomalies in the MRI had histologically confirmed hippocampal sclerosis [80]. However, exact focus localization is not guaranteed with either of these PET techniques.

Neuropsychological Testing

Thorough neuropsychological evaluation is essential because it can reveal cognitive deficits, typically referring to memory functions pointing to hippocampal damage. Most patients have neuropsychological deficits that correctly lateralize to the side of seizure focus [50]. According to the literature, neuropsychological testing is probably more sensitive in detecting left-sided than right-sided abnormalities [50]. Furthermore, neuropsychological testing is an important part of presurgical epilepsy evaluation. It can provide clues as to how much function is retained in the affected hippocampus and thus what the patient is expected to lose after hippocampectomy. This is especially crucial in patients with hippocampal sclerosis of the dominant hemisphere, as epilepsy surgery in the temporal lobe of the language-dominant hemisphere has been shown to bear the risk of verbal memory decline [81].

The most typical type of neuropsychological deficit in MTLE-HS is impairment of long-term memory consolidation or retrieval of newly acquired information [1]. Other cognitive deficits, like impairment of material-specific and verbal memory are less specific and also depend on whether the epileptogenic focus is located in the language-dominant hemisphere or not. The grade of memory dysfunction is influenced by several parameters: frequency and severity of seizures, age of onset of epilepsy, medication, mental reserve capacity, and degree of atrophy of the hippocampus [1, 82–86]. It is often suggested that high-frequency seizures or severe and longer seizures may lead to progression of neuropsychological deficits. The severity of memory decline over time depends on many parameters and is not yet completely clear. Cross-sectional studies show a stronger effect than the longitudinal ones, which showed a definite (albeit mild) relationship between epilepsy and memory decline [87].

Presurgical evaluation should include lateralization of language function. Nowadays, this is usually done by fMRI. In some cases, an intracarotid amobarbital test (Wada test) is used to lateralize language and to determine the memory function potential of the hippocampus contralateral to the planned surgery [50]. However, it has been shown that this rather invasive test is not superior to a combined thorough evaluation with neuropsychological testing and fMRI.

Therapeutic Management, Risks, and Prognosis

Antiepileptic Medication
As with all epilepsies, the typical procedure is to first try an anticonvulsive treatment. The usual consensus is that the epilepsy is declared as medically refractory if seizures persist despite adequate treatment with two consecutive first-line antiepileptic drugs [88]. Epilepsies with focal seizures and temporal lobe abnormalities like hippocampal sclerosis are often drug resistant (in up to 70% of cases), more often than in other MRI-identified lesions [1, 89–91].

Epilepsy Surgery
In these medically refractory cases, epilepsy surgery is considered. Because of the good efficacy of epilepsy surgery in this particular case, it is nowadays increasingly common to refer patients to a resective treatment quite early, although some patients may of course become seizure-free with multiple antiepileptic drugs or – in very rare cases – even without treatment [92]. While the numbers seem to have decreased in the last years, temporal lobe epilepsy with hippocampal sclerosis is the type of epilepsy most frequently operated on [93]. There are various major temporal lobe surgeries: standard anterior temporal lobectomy, electrocorticography-guided temporal lobectomy, and anteromedial temporal lobectomy [94]. There is evidence for a total and against a partial hippocampectomy [92, 95]. The parahippocampal gyrus and the amygdala are generally removed along with the hippocampus, as studies have shown that they play an important role in generating and propagating seizures [92, 96].

Almost all epilepsy surgery procedures in patients with hippocampal sclerosis involve not only the resection of the hippocampus, but also of adjacent structures [97, 98], including temporal lobectomy in some cases. In patients in which ictal activity is definitely localized in the hippocampus, selective (transcortical, transsylvian, or subtemporal) amygdalohippocampectomy can be performed [94]. In a few cases, hippocampal transection has been reported with the aim to reduce postoperative memory deficits in the dominant hemisphere [94, 99, 100]. Stereotactic amygdalohippocampectomy has been performed in some patients, but this is not a standard procedure [94, 101–103].

The goal of surgery is to achieve seizure freedom while preserving as much cognitive function as possible. Which resection method gives the best seizure outcome remains a subject of debate [104].

Epilepsy Surgery Risks
Complications from epilepsy surgery in the temporal lobe vary in features and frequency. Apart from general surgical complications such as hemorrhage and infection, there are specific risks for this kind of resective surgery. Probably the most common neurological deficit following temporal lobe surgery is a contralateral superior qua-

drantanopsia caused by damage to the optic radiation fibers in the roof of the temporal horn [92, 94, 105], even if restrictive selective resections are performed [106]. In most cases, patients are not aware of this quadrantanopsia because fortunately it does not hinder them in everyday life [105]. Depending on the part of the optic radiation injured, visual field deficits vary between small defects to (rarely) homonymous hemianopsia.

Postoperative memory deficits are a much-feared complication of temporal lobe surgery with resection of the hippocampus, even in carefully selected patients with neuropsychological, fMRI, and/or Wada testing. As the hippocampus plays an important role in visuospatial (nondominant hemisphere) and verbal (dominant hemisphere) memory, as well as in long-term memory, these functions are most commonly compromised [81, 92]. Temporal lobe resections in the dominant hemisphere can cause a decline in verbal memory, even if the hippocampus is not resected. However, hippocampus-sparing surgery has been shown to be associated with a benefit in verbal learning [81, 107, 108]. Due to the high probability of memory deficits, epilepsy surgery in this region should be considered extremely carefully in patients with good ipsilateral memory function as well as in patients with relevant contralateral hippocampal dysfunction because bilateral hippocampal damage is known to cause severe amnesia, as in the famous case of Henry Molaison [109].

Temporal lobe surgery in the dominant hemisphere bears the risk of language deficits because of the localization of Broca's (interior frontal gyrus) and Wernicke's area (posterior superior temporal gyrus) and their involvement due to direct injury, brain retraction, deafferentation, ischemia, or edema [92, 94, 110, 111]. The most common manifestations are dysphasia and dysnomia (about 30%), of which the majority are transient [92, 94, 112–116]. In some centers, language mapping by electrical stimulation is preoperatively performed in patients with intracranial EEG electrodes, or intraoperative language mapping is performed to define the borders of resection [115, 116]. There is evidence, however, that the latter method does not significantly prevent language deficits [113, 115, 116].

Patients with temporal lobe epilepsy often demonstrate psychiatric comorbidity, especially depression (up to 74% of cases), anxiety disorders (up to 25%), psychoses (up to 9%), and personality disorders (about 2%) [117]. In most cases, these psychiatric disorders, particularly the depression, improve postsurgically, following a remission of the epilepsy. Some patients (less than 10% in the literature), however, develop psychiatric disorders, mostly depression but also psychosis, after surgery. Presurgical depression or psychosis and epileptiform discharges contralateral to the epileptogenic zone are described as risk factors associated with postsurgical psychiatric morbidity [117, 118].

Motor deficits like hemiparesis are quite uncommon (less than 2%), but are possible, usually as a result of injury or thrombosis of the anterior choroidal artery [94, 119]. Cranial nerve injury (oculomotor, trochlear, and facial nerves), most often caused by traction, is not very frequent (up to 3%) and usually transient [92, 119].

Epilepsy Surgery Results and Prognosis

The majority (over 80%) of patients who become seizure-free after temporal lobectomy have hippocampal sclerosis as their main pathology [8]. Although there is a robust association between postoperative seizure freedom and resection of the abnormal hippocampus and some studies have suggested that hippocampal sclerosis on MRI is a predictor of good outcome after surgery [104, 120, 121], data suggest that other temporal structures may play a role in the epileptic network, even when the primary pathology lies in the hippocampus itself. Case series, reviews of observational studies, and controlled trials have demonstrated the short- and long-term efficacy of temporal lobe resection and amygdalohippocampectomy in the treatment of mesial temporal epilepsy.

In a randomized, controlled trial comparing epilepsy surgery with medical treatment for temporal lobe epilepsy, 58% of the patients in the surgical group were without disabling seizures, compared with 8% free from disabling seizures in the medical treatment group [105].

Another randomized trial compared selective amygdalohippocampectomy with medical treatment. In a mean follow-up of about 26 months, antiepileptic medication use and seizure frequency were significantly reduced after this surgical procedure – 82% of patients became seizure free [122]. Similarly positive results have been shown in other studies with amygdalohippocampectomy alone (about 60% seizure freedom) [123] or in combination with temporal lobectomy (84% of patients in Engel class[1] I or II) [104], or with anterior temporal lobectomy (89% seizure free, 94% Engel class I or II) [126]. These positive effects have been shown to be stable over a long period of time. In a long-term outcome study with temporal lobe epilepsy surgery, the percentage of patients still in Engel class I after 16 years was about 70% [120].

The hippocampus plays an important role in this context, as signs of hippocampal sclerosis and/or atrophy on the preoperative MRI have often been shown to be a predictor for a positive outcome after surgery [120, 121, 127, 128]. However, many authors point out that concordant EEG, video-EEG monitoring, and neuropsychological data are important in predicting outcome as well [127]. Further predictors of positive outcome are febrile seizures and early surgery [121, 127–129]. Negative predictors are bilateral interictal sharp waves, necessity of intracranial EEG recording, and multiple seizure types [120, 127, 130, 131].

Surgical outcome in children with hippocampal sclerosis is similar to that in adults, although MRI may not be as sensitive as in older patients [131]. Negative outcome predictors include multiple seizure types, developmental delay, multifocal EEG abnormalities, and high seizure frequency [131].

---

[1] Epilepsy surgery outcome according to the Engel classification [124, 125]: class I: free of disabling seizures, class II: rare disabling seizures, class III: worthwhile improvement, class IV: no worthwhile improvement.

Neuropsychological and Psychiatric Outcomes

Due to the important role the hippocampus plays in memory and learning, mesial temporal resections bear the risk of postoperative memory deficits. While bilateral hippocampal damage causes serious anterograde amnesia, unilateral damage does not necessarily lead to severe memory dysfunction, provided the contralateral hippocampus is intact. This emphasizes the importance of neuropsychological and functional examinations (Wada test, fMRI, PET) in the preoperative evaluation. However, it has been demonstrated that learning and recall of words is impaired in patients with resections (irrespective of type) of the left temporal lobe, while right temporal surgery did not lead to memory impairment [108]. Verbal memory is the most systematically affected, particularly in surgery of the language-dominant hemisphere [132]. The memory reserve capacity and thus the postoperative memory outcome can be assessed by using the following parameters: baseline performance (patients with high preoperative memory scores are at greatest risk of postoperative memory decline), functional adequacy of resected tissue, and seizure outcome [1, 133]. Although verbal memory decline has been observed after left temporal resections in long-term follow-up evaluation, there has also been a trend for contralateral improvement of nonverbal memory [1, 132]. There have been comparisons of different surgery types regarding the postoperative cognitive outcome, assuming that more selective surgery procedures could bear a lower risk for memory deficits [1, 134, 135]. There is evidence that highly selective surgery, like selective amygdalohippocampectomy, leads to better neuropsychological results [136]. It is also known that while temporal lobe resections within the language-dominant hemisphere can cause verbal memory decline even if the hippocampus is spared, hippocampus-sparing surgery (for selected patients) is associated with a benefit in verbal learning performance.

Depression and anxiety are common psychiatric disorders in patients with epilepsy. Available data from a large prospective study (360 patients, 89% with temporal lobectomy) show a significantly decline of depression and anxiety over a follow-up period of 2 years [137]. In general, the psychosocial outcome after epilepsy surgery appears to be linked to a change in self and a transition from chronically illness to health [138].

Stereotactic Radiofrequency Amygdalohippocampectomy

Stereotactic radiosurgery of the hippocampus has been suggested as an alternative to conventional surgery in order to minimize complications. Two pilot trials as well as case reports have shown the efficacy of this procedure, with approximately 65–77% of patients achieving seizure freedom [139–141]. However, damage to the surrounding cerebral tissue is possible (and even delayed) and data for long-term follow-up are scarce [142–146].

Hippocampal Stimulation (and Other Brain Stimulation)

Because of the invasive nature of epilepsy surgery and the fact that quite a few patients are not suitable for this treatment or do not show adequate postoperative seizure control, there is strong interest in brain stimulation for the treatment of epilepsy. The advantages of brain stimulation are self-explanatory. Being less invasive than, for example, amygdalohippocampectomy or temporal lobe resection, there should be a decreased risk of causing neuropsychological or visual deficits. Furthermore, stimulation can be stopped if needed, rendering possible side effects reversible. Hippocampal stimulation has been explored in the treatment of mesial temporal epilepsy. The mechanisms involved remain unclear, although there have been suggestions that activation of perforant pathway fibers results in polysynaptic inhibition of epileptogenic neurons [147]. Some case series and small double-blind studies have investigated the use of hippocampal stimulation (in some cases unilateral, in other bilateral) in the treatment of patients with mesial temporal epilepsy [147–149]. Electrodes were placed along the axis of the hippocampi. Seizure freedom or significant seizure reduction was achieved in most of the patients, while adverse effects were reported to be practically absent [148–151]. These are encouraging results that need to be confirmed in larger randomized controlled trials, like the ongoing CoRaStir study (http://clinicaltrials.gov/ct2/show/NCT00431457).

References

1 Wieser HG: ILAE Commission Report. Mesial temporal lobe epilepsy with hippocampal sclerosis. Epilepsia 2004;45:695–714.

2 Gil-Nagel A, Risinger MW: Ictal semiology in hippocampal versus extrahippocampal temporal lobe epilepsy. Brain 1997;120:183–192.

3 Mathern GW, Pretorius JK, Babb TL: Influence of the type of initial precipitating injury and at what age it occurs on course and outcome in patients with temporal lobe seizures. J Neurosurg 1995;82:220–227.

4 Mathern GW, Leite JP, Pretorius JK, Quinn B, Peacock WJ, Babb TL: Severe seizures in young children are associated with hippocampal neuron losses and aberrant mossy fiber sprouting during fascia dentata postnatal development. Epilepsy Res Suppl 1996;12:33–43.

5 Berg AT, Langfitt J, Shinnar S, Vickrey BG, Sperling MR, Walczak T, Bazil C, Pacia SV, Spencer SS: How long does it take for partial epilepsy to become intractable? Neurology 2003;60:186–190.

6 Berg AT, Berkovic SF, Brodie MJ, Buchhalter J, Cross JH, van Emde Boas W, Engel J, French J, Glauser TA, Mathern GW, Moshe SL, Nordli D, Plouin P, Scheffer IE: Revised terminology and concepts for organization of seizures and epilepsies: report of the ILAE Commission on Classification and Terminology, 2005–2009. Epilepsia 2010;51:676–685.

7 Blair RG: Temporal lobe epilepsy semiology. Epilepsy Res Treat 2012;2012:751510.

8 French JA, Williamson PD, Thadani VM, Darcey TM, Mattson RH, Spencer SS, Spencer DD: Characteristics of medial temporal lobe epilepsy: I. Results of history and physical examination. Ann Neurol 1993;34:774–780.

9 Henkel A, Noachtar S, Pfander M, Luders HO: The localizing value of the abdominal aura and its evolution: a study in focal epilepsies. Neurology 2002;58:271–276.

10 Pfander M, Arnold S, Henkel A, Weil S, Werhahn KJ, Eisensehr I, Winkler PA, Noachtar S: Clinical features and EEG findings differentiating mesial from neocortical temporal lobe epilepsy. Epileptic Disord 2002;4:189–195.

11 Ray A, Kotagal P: Temporal lobe epilepsy in children: overview of clinical semiology. Epileptic Disord 2005;7:299–307.

12 Fried I, Spencer DD, Spencer SS: The anatomy of epileptic auras: focal pathology and surgical outcome. J Neurosurg 1995;83:60–66.

13 Lieb JP, Dasheiff RM, Engel JJ: Role of the frontal lobes in the propagation of mesial temporal lobe seizures. Epilepsia 1991;32:822–837.

14 Lothman EW, Bertram EH 3rd, Stringer JL: Functional anatomy of hippocampal seizures. Prog Neurobiol 1991;37:1–82.

15 Lothman EW: Seizure circuits in the hippocampus and associated structures. Hippocampus 1994;4:286–290.

16 Foldvary-Schaefer N, Unnwongse K: Localizing and lateralizing features of auras and seizures. Epilepsy Behav 2011;20:160–166.

17 Loddenkemper T, Kellinghaus C, Gandjour J, Nair DR, Najm IM, Bingaman W, Luders HO: Localising and lateralising value of ictal piloerection. J Neurol Neurosurg Psychiatry 2004;75:879–883.

18 Margerison JH, Corsellis JA: Epilepsy and the temporal lobes. A clinical, electroencephalographic and neuropathological study of the brain in epilepsy, with particular reference to the temporal lobes. Brain 1966;89:499–530.

19 Annegers JF, Hauser WA, Elveback LR, Kurland LT: The risk of epilepsy following febrile convulsions. Neurology 1979;29:297–303.

20 Berg AT: The natural history of mesial temporal lobe epilepsy. Curr Opin Neurol 2008;21:173–178.

21 Ellenberg JH, Nelson KB: Febrile seizures and later intellectual performance. Arch Neurol 1978;35:17–21.

22 Scott RC, King MD, Gadian DG, Neville BG, Connelly A: Hippocampal abnormalities after prolonged febrile convulsion: a longitudinal MRI study. Brain 2003;126:2551–2557.

23 Thom M: Recent advances in the neuropathology of focal lesions in epilepsy. Expert Rev Neurother 2004; 4:973–984.

24 Kunz WS, Kudin AP, Vielhaber S, Blumcke I, Zuschratter W, Schramm J, Beck H, Elger CE: Mitochondrial complex I deficiency in the epileptic focus of patients with temporal lobe epilepsy. Ann Neurol 2000;48:766–773.

25 Crespel A, Coubes P, Rousset MC, Brana C, Rougier A, Rondouin G, Bockaert J, Baldy-Moulinier M, Lerner-Natoli M: Inflammatory reactions in human medial temporal lobe epilepsy with hippocampal sclerosis. Brain Res 2002;952:159–169.

26 Blumcke I, Thom M, Wiestler OD: Ammon's horn sclerosis: a maldevelopmental disorder associated with temporal lobe epilepsy. Brain Pathol 2002;12:199–211.

27 Cendes F, Lopes-Cendes I, Andermann E, Andermann F: Familial temporal lobe epilepsy: a clinically heterogeneous syndrome. Neurology 1998;50:554–557.

28 Kobayashi E, Li LM, Lopes-Cendes I, Cendes F: Magnetic resonance imaging evidence of hippocampal sclerosis in asymptomatic, first-degree relatives of patients with familial mesial temporal lobe epilepsy. Arch Neurol 2002;59:1891–1894.

29 Fisher PD, Sperber EF, Moshe SL: Hippocampal sclerosis revisited. Brain Dev 1998;20:563–573.

30 Sloviter RS: Decreased hippocampal inhibition and a selective loss of interneurons in experimental epilepsy. Science 1987;235:73–76.

31 Sloviter RS: On the relationship between neuropathology and pathophysiology in the epileptic hippocampus of humans and experimental animals. Hippocampus 1994;4:250–253.

32 Nadler JV, Perry BW, Cotman CW: Selective reinnervation of hippocampal area CA1 and the fascia dentata after destruction of CA3-CA4 afferents with kainic acid. Brain Res 1980;182:1–9.

33 Tauck DL, Nadler JV: Evidence of functional mossy fiber sprouting in hippocampal formation of kainic acid-treated rats. J Neurosci 1985;5:1016–1022.

34 Franck JE, Pokorny J, Kunkel DD, Schwartzkroin PA: Physiologic and morphologic characteristics of granule cell circuitry in human epileptic hippocampus. Epilepsia 1995;36:543–558.

35 Coulter DA, McIntyre DC, Loscher W: Animal models of limbic epilepsies: what can they tell us? Brain Pathol 2002;12:240–256.

36 Cronin J, Dudek FE: Chronic seizures and collateral sprouting of dentate mossy fibers after kainic acid treatment in rats. Brain Res 1988;474:181–184.

37 Cavazos JE, Sutula TP: Progressive neuronal loss induced by kindling: a possible mechanism for mossy fiber synaptic reorganization and hippocampal sclerosis. Brain Res 1990;527:1–6.

38 Chatzikonstantinou A, Gass A, Forster A, Hennerici MG, Szabo K: Features of acute DWI abnormalities related to status epilepticus. Epilepsy Res 2011;97:45–51.

39 Provenzale JM, Liang L, DeLong D, White LE: Diffusion tensor imaging assessment of brain white matter maturation during the first postnatal year. AJR Am J Roentgenol 2007;189:476–486.

40 Araujo D, Santos AC, Velasco TR, Wichert-Ana L, Terra-Bustamante VC, Alexandre VJ, Carlotti CGJ, Assirati JAJ, Machado HR, Walz R, Leite JP, Sakamoto AC: Volumetric evidence of bilateral damage in unilateral mesial temporal lobe epilepsy. Epilepsia 2006;47:1354–1359.

41 Jokeit H, Ebner A, Arnold S, Schuller M, Antke C, Huang Y, Steinmetz H, Seitz RJ, Witte OW: Bilateral reductions of hippocampal volume, glucose metabolism, and wada hemispheric memory performance are related to the duration of mesial temporal lobe epilepsy. J Neurol 1999;246:926–933.

42 Cendes F, Andermann F, Gloor P, Lopes-Cendes I, Andermann E, Melanson D, Jones-Gotman M, Robitaille Y, Evans A, Peters T: Atrophy of mesial structures in patients with temporal lobe epilepsy: cause or consequence of repeated seizures? Ann Neurol 1993;34:795–801.

43 Lado FA, Laureta EC, Moshe SL: Seizure-induced hippocampal damage in the mature and immature brain. Epileptic Disord 2002;4:83–97.

44 Thom M, Zhou J, Martinian L, Sisodiya S: Quantitative post-mortem study of the hippocampus in chronic epilepsy: seizures do not inevitably cause neuronal loss. Brain 2005;128:1344–1357.

45 Salmenpera T, Kononen M, Roberts N, Vanninen R, Pitkanen A, Kalviainen R: Hippocampal damage in newly diagnosed focal epilepsy: a prospective MRI study. Neurology 2005;64:62–68.

46 Van Paesschen W, Duncan JS, Stevens JM, Connelly A: Longitudinal quantitative hippocampal magnetic resonance imaging study of adults with newly diagnosed partial seizures: one-year follow-up results. Epilepsia 1998;39:633–639.

47 Kasper BS, Stefan H, Buchfelder M, Paulus W: Temporal lobe microdysgenesis in epilepsy versus control brains. J Neuropathol Exp Neurol 1999;58:22–28.

48 Yilmazer-Hanke DM, Wolf HK, Schramm J, Elger CE, Wiestler OD, Blumcke I: Subregional pathology of the amygdala complex and entorhinal region in surgical specimens from patients with pharmacoresistant temporal lobe epilepsy. J Neuropathol Exp Neurol 2000;59:907–920.

49 Koutroumanidis M, Binnie CD, Elwes RD, Polkey CE, Seed P, Alarcon G, Cox T, Barrington S, Marsden P, Maisey MN, Panayiotopoulos CP: Interictal regional slow activity in temporal lobe epilepsy correlates with lateral temporal hypometabolism as imaged with ^{18}FDG PET: neurophysiological and metabolic implications. J Neurol Neurosurg Psychiatry 1998;65:170–176.

50 Williamson PD, French JA, Thadani VM, Kim JH, Novelly RA, Spencer SS, Spencer DD, Mattson RH: Characteristics of medial temporal lobe epilepsy: II. Interictal and ictal scalp electroencephalography, neuropsychological testing, neuroimaging, surgical results, and pathology. Ann Neurol 1993;34:781–787.

51 Risinger MW, Engel JJ, Van Ness PC, Henry TR, Crandall PH: Ictal localization of temporal lobe seizures with scalp/sphenoidal recordings. Neurology 1989;39:1288–1293.

52 King D, Spencer S: Invasive electroencephalography in mesial temporal lobe epilepsy. J Clin Neurophysiol 1995;12:32–45.

53 King D, Spencer SS, McCarthy G, Spencer DD: Surface and depth EEG findings in patients with hippocampal atrophy. Neurology 1997;48:1363–1367.

54 Berkovic SF, Andermann F, Olivier A, Ethier R, Melanson D, Robitaille Y, Kuzniecky R, Peters T, Feindel W: Hippocampal sclerosis in temporal lobe epilepsy demonstrated by magnetic resonance imaging. Ann Neurol 1991;29:175–182.

55 Jackson GD, Berkovic SF, Tress BM, Kalnins RM, Fabinyi GC, Bladin PF: Hippocampal sclerosis can be reliably detected by magnetic resonance imaging. Neurology 1990;40:1869–1875.

56 Henry TR, Chupin M, Lehericy S, Strupp JP, Sikora MA, Sha ZY, Ugurbil K, Van de Moortele PF: Hippocampal sclerosis in temporal lobe epilepsy: findings at 7 T(1). Radiology 2011;261:199–209.

57 Jack CR: MRI-based hippocampal volume measurements in epilepsy. Epilepsia 1994;35(suppl 6):S21–S29.

58 Jafari-Khouzani K, Elisevich K, Patel S, Smith B, Soltanian-Zadeh H: FLAIR signal and texture analysis for lateralizing mesial temporal lobe epilepsy. Neuroimage 2010;49:1559–1571.

59 Bronen RA, Cheung G, Charles JT, Kim JH, Spencer DD, Spencer SS, Sze G, McCarthy G: Imaging findings in hippocampal sclerosis: correlation with pathology. AJNR Am J Neuroradiol 1991;12:933–940.

60 Van Paesschen W, Revesz T, Duncan JS, King MD, Connelly A: Quantitative neuropathology and quantitative magnetic resonance imaging of the hippocampus in temporal lobe epilepsy. Ann Neurol 1997;42:756–766.

61 Pardoe HR, Pell GS, Abbott DF, Jackson GD: Hippocampal volume assessment in temporal lobe epilepsy: how good is automated segmentation? Epilepsia 2009;50:2586–2592.

62 Malmgren K, Thom M: Hippocampal sclerosis – origins and imaging. Epilepsia 2012;53(suppl 4):19–33.

63 Moran NF, Lemieux L, Kitchen ND, Fish DR, Shorvon SD: Extrahippocampal temporal lobe atrophy in temporal lobe epilepsy and mesial temporal sclerosis. Brain 2001;124:167–175.

64 Hofman PA, Fitt G, Mitchell LA, Jackson GD: Hippocampal sclerosis and a second focal lesion – how often is it ipsilateral? Epilepsia 2011;52:718–721.

65 Menzler K, Iwinska-Zelder J, Shiratori K, Jaeger RK, Oertel WH, Hamer HM, Rosenow F, Knake S: Evaluation of MRI criteria (1.5 T) for the diagnosis of hippocampal sclerosis in healthy subjects. Epilepsy Res 2010;89:349–354.

66 Labate A, Gambardella A, Aguglia U, Condino F, Ventura P, Lanza P, Quattrone A: Temporal lobe abnormalities on brain MRI in healthy volunteers: a prospective case-control study. Neurology 2010;74:553–557.

67 Hashiguchi K, Morioka T, Murakami N, Suzuki SO, Hiwatashi A, Yoshiura T, Sasaki T: Utility of 3-T FLAIR and 3D short tau inversion recovery MR imaging in the preoperative diagnosis of hippocampal sclerosis: direct comparison with 1.5-T FLAIR MR imaging. Epilepsia 2010;51:1820–1828.

68 Von Oertzen J, Urbach H, Jungbluth S, Kurthen M, Reuber M, Fernandez G, Elger CE: Standard magnetic resonance imaging is inadequate for patients with refractory focal epilepsy. J Neurol Neurosurg Psychiatry 2002;73:643–647.

69 Cendes F, Andermann F, Preul MC, Arnold DL: Lateralization of temporal lobe epilepsy based on regional metabolic abnormalities in proton magnetic resonance spectroscopic images. Ann Neurol 1994;35:211–216.

70 Woermann FG, McLean MA, Bartlett PA, Parker GJ, Barker GJ, Duncan JS: Short echo time single-voxel ^{1}H magnetic resonance spectroscopy in magnetic resonance imaging-negative temporal lobe epilepsy: different biochemical profile compared with hippocampal sclerosis. Ann Neurol 1999;45:369–376.

Chatzikonstantinou

71 Willmann O, Wennberg R, May T, Woermann FG, Pohlmann-Eden B: The role of ^{1}H magnetic resonance spectroscopy in pre-operative evaluation for epilepsy surgery. A meta-analysis. Epilepsy Res 2006; 71:149–158.

72 Cendes F, Andermann F, Dubeau F, Arnold DL: Proton magnetic resonance spectroscopic images and MRI volumetric studies for lateralization of temporal lobe epilepsy. Magn Reson Imaging 1995;13: 1187–1191.

73 Bonnici HM, Sidhu M, Chadwick MJ, Duncan JS, Maguire EA: Assessing hippocampal functional reserve in temporal lobe epilepsy: a multi-voxel pattern analysis of fMRI data. Epilepsy Res 2013;105:140–149.

74 Engel JJ, Henry TR, Risinger MW, Mazziotta JC, Sutherling WW, Levesque MF, Phelps ME: Presurgical evaluation for partial epilepsy: relative contributions of chronic depth-electrode recordings versus FDG-PET and scalp-sphenoidal ictal EEG. Neurology 1990;40:1670–1677.

75 Henry TR, Sutherling WW, Engel JJ, Risinger MW, Levesque MF, Mazziotta JC, Phelps ME: Interictal cerebral metabolism in partial epilepsies of neocortical origin. Epilepsy Res 1991;10:174–182.

76 Chassoux F, Semah F, Bouilleret V, Landre E, Devaux B, Turak B, Nataf F, Roux FX: Metabolic changes and electro-clinical patterns in mesio-temporal lobe epilepsy: a correlative study. Brain 2004; 127:164–174.

77 Knowlton RC, Laxer KD, Klein G, Sawrie S, Ende G, Hawkins RA, Aassar OS, Soohoo K, Wong S, Barbaro N: In vivo hippocampal glucose metabolism in mesial temporal lobe epilepsy. Neurology 2001;57: 1184–1190.

78 Semah F, Baulac M, Hasboun D, Frouin V, Mangin JF, Papageorgiou S, Leroy-Willig A, Philippon J, Laplane D, Samson Y: Is interictal temporal hypometabolism related to mesial temporal sclerosis? A positron emission tomography/magnetic resonance imaging confrontation. Epilepsia 1995;36:447–456.

79 Willmann O, Wennberg R, May T, Woermann FG, Pohlmann-Eden B: The contribution of ^{18}F-FDG PET in preoperative epilepsy surgery evaluation for patients with temporal lobe epilepsy. A meta-analysis. Seizure 2007;16:509–520.

80 Lamusuo S, Pitkanen A, Jutila L, Ylinen A, Partanen K, Kalviainen R, Ruottinen HM, Oikonen V, Nagren K, Lehikoinen P, Vapalahti M, Vainio P, Rinne JO: [11 C]Flumazenil binding in the medial temporal lobe in patients with temporal lobe epilepsy: correlation with hippocampal MR volumetry, T2 relaxometry, and neuropathology. Neurology 2000;54:2252–2260.

81 Wagner K, Uherek M, Horstmann S, Kadish NE, Wisniewski I, Mayer H, Buschmann F, Metternich B, Zentner J, Schulze-Bonhage A: Memory outcome after hippocampus sparing resections in the temporal lobe. J Neurol Neurosurg Psychiatry 2013;84:630–636.

82 Baxendale SA, Van Paesschen W, Thompson PJ, Duncan JS, Harkness WF, Shorvon SD: Hippocampal cell loss and gliosis: relationship to preoperative and postoperative memory function. Neuropsychiatry Neuropsychol Behav Neurol 1998;11: 12–21.

83 Baxendale SA, van Paesschen W, Thompson PJ, Connelly A, Duncan JS, Harkness WF, Shorvon SD: The relationship between quantitative MRI and neuropsychological functioning in temporal lobe epilepsy. Epilepsia 1998;39:158–166.

84 Hermann BP, Wyler AR, Richey ET: Wisconsin Card Sorting Test performance in patients with complex partial seizures of temporal-lobe origin. J Clin Exp Neuropsychol 1988;10:467–476.

85 Jokeit H, Seitz RJ, Markowitsch HJ, Neumann N, Witte OW, Ebner A: Prefrontal asymmetric interictal glucose hypometabolism and cognitive impairment in patients with temporal lobe epilepsy. Brain 1997;120:2283–2294.

86 Sawrie SM, Martin RC, Knowlton R, Faught E, Gilliam F, Kuzniecky R: Relationships among hippocampal volumetry, proton magnetic resonance spectroscopy, and verbal memory in temporal lobe epilepsy. Epilepsia 2001;42:1403–1407.

87 Dodrill CB: Progressive cognitive decline in adolescents and adults with epilepsy. Prog Brain Res 2002; 135:399–407.

88 Engel JJ, Wiebe S, French J, Sperling M, Williamson P, Spencer D, Gumnit R, Zahn C, Westbrook E, Enos B: Practice parameter: temporal lobe and localized neocortical resections for epilepsy: report of the Quality Standards Subcommittee of the American Academy of Neurology, in association with the American Epilepsy Society and the American Association of Neurological Surgeons. Neurology 2003; 60:538–547.

89 Josephson CB, Pohlmann-Eden B: The 'natural' history of medically treated temporal lobe epilepsy: what can an evidence-based approach tell us? Epilepsy Res Treat 2012;2012:216510.

90 Mattson RH, Cramer JA, Collins JF: Prognosis for total control of complex partial and secondarily generalized tonic clonic seizures. Department of Veterans Affairs Epilepsy Cooperative Studies No. 118 and No. 264 Group. Neurology 1996;47:68–76.

91 Semah F, Picot MC, Adam C, Broglin D, Arzimanoglou A, Bazin B, Cavalcanti D, Baulac M: Is the underlying cause of epilepsy a major prognostic factor for recurrence? Neurology 1998;51:1256–1262.

92 Mansouri A, Fallah A, Valiante TA: Determining surgical candidacy in temporal lobe epilepsy. Epilepsy Res Treat 2012;2012:706917.

93 Janszky J, Janszky I, Schulz R, Hoppe M, Behne F, Pannek HW, Ebner A: Temporal lobe epilepsy with hippocampal sclerosis: predictors for long-term surgical outcome. Brain 2005;128:395–404.

94 Al-Otaibi F, Baeesa SS, Parrent AG, Girvin JP, Steven D: Surgical techniques for the treatment of temporal lobe epilepsy. Epilepsy Res Treat 2012; 2012:374848.

95 Wyler AR, Hermann BP, Somes G: Extent of medial temporal resection on outcome from anterior temporal lobectomy: a randomized prospective study. Neurosurgery 1995;37:982–990, discussion 990–991.

96 Wennberg R, Arruda F, Quesney LF, Olivier A: Preeminence of extrahippocampal structures in the generation of mesial temporal seizures: evidence from human depth electrode recordings. Epilepsia 2002;43:716–726.

97 Falconer MA: Surgical treatment of temporal lobe epilepsy. NZ Med J 1967;66:539–542.

98 Spencer DD, Spencer SS, Mattson RH, Williamson PD, Novelly RA: Access to the posterior medial temporal lobe structures in the surgical treatment of temporal lobe epilepsy. Neurosurgery 1984;15:667–671.

99 Shimizu H, Kawai K, Sunaga S, Sugano H, Yamada T: Hippocampal transection for treatment of left temporal lobe epilepsy with preservation of verbal memory. J Clin Neurosci 2006;13:322–328.

100 Sunaga S, Morino M, Kusakabe T, Sugano H, Shimizu H: Efficacy of hippocampal transection for left temporal lobe epilepsy without hippocampal atrophy. Epilepsy Behav 2011;21:94–99.

101 Kitchen ND, Thomas DG, Thompson PJ, Shorvon SD, Fish DR: Open stereotactic amygdalohippocampectomy – clinical, psychometric, and MRI follow-up. Acta Neurochir (Wien) 1993;123:33–38.

102 Miyagi Y, Shima F, Ishido K, Araki T, Taniwaki Y, Okamoto I, Kamikaseda K: Inferior temporal sulcus approach for amygdalohippocampectomy guided by a laser beam of stereotactic navigator. Neurosurgery 2003; 52: 1117–1123, discussion 1123–1124.

103 Parrent AG, Blume WT: Stereotactic amygdalohippocampotomy for the treatment of medial temporal lobe epilepsy. Epilepsia 1999;40:1408–1416.

104 Vadera S, Kshettry VR, Klaas P, Bingaman W: Seizure-free and neuropsychological outcomes after temporal lobectomy with amygdalohippocampectomy in pediatric patients with hippocampal sclerosis. J Neurosurg Pediatr 2012;10:103–107.

105 Wiebe S, Blume WT, Girvin JP, Eliasziw M: A randomized, controlled trial of surgery for temporal-lobe epilepsy. N Engl J Med 2001;345:311–318.

106 Egan RA, Shults WT, So N, Burchiel K, Kellogg JX, Salinsky M: Visual field deficits in conventional anterior temporal lobectomy versus amygdalohippocampectomy. Neurology 2000;55:1818–1822.

107 Elsharkawy AE, Pannek H, Woermann FG, Gyimesi C, Hartmann S, Aengenendt J, Ogutu T, Hoppe M, Schulz R, Pietila TA, Ebner A: Apical temporal lobe resection; 'tailored' hippocampus-sparing resection based on presurgical evaluation data. Acta Neurochir (Wien) 2011;153:231–238.

108 Jones-Gotman M, Zatorre RJ, Olivier A, Andermann F, Cendes F, Staunton H, McMackin D, Siegel AM, Wieser HG: Learning and retention of words and designs following excision from medial or lateral temporal-lobe structures. Neuropsychologia 1997;35:963–973.

109 Scoville WB, Milner B: Loss of recent memory after bilateral hippocampal lesions. J Neurol Neurosurg Psychiatry 1957;20:11–21.

110 Helgason CM, Bergen D, Bleck TP, Morrell F, Whisler W: Infarction after surgery for focal epilepsy: manipulation hemiplegia revisited. Epilepsia 1987;28:340–345.

111 Penfield W: Pitfalls and success in surgical treatment of focal epilepsy. Br Med J 1958;1:669–672.

112 Davies KG, Risse GL, Gates JR: Naming ability after tailored left temporal resection with extraoperative language mapping: increased risk of decline with later epilepsy onset age. Epilepsy Behav 2005;7:273–278.

113 Hermann BP, Perrine K, Chelune GJ, Barr W, Loring DW, Strauss E, Trenerry MR, Westerveld M: Visual confrontation naming following left anterior temporal lobectomy: a comparison of surgical approaches. Neuropsychology 1999;13:3–9.

114 Pilcher WH, Rusyniak WG: Complications of epilepsy surgery. Neurosurg Clin N Am 1993;4:311–325.

115 Stafiniak P, Saykin AJ, Sperling MR, Kester DB, Robinson LJ, O'Connor MJ, Gur RC: Acute naming deficits following dominant temporal lobectomy: prediction by age at 1st risk for seizures. Neurology 1990;40:1509–1512.

116 Wyllie E, Luders H, Morris HH 3rd, Lesser RP, Dinner DS, Hahn J, Estes ML, Rothner AD, Erenberg G, Cruse R, et al: Clinical outcome after complete or partial cortical resection for intractable epilepsy. Neurology 1987;37:1634–1641.

117 Filho GM, Mazetto L, Gomes FL, Marinho MM, Tavares IM, Caboclo LO, Centeno RS, Yacubian EM: Pre-surgical predictors for psychiatric disorders following epilepsy surgery in patients with refractory temporal lobe epilepsy and mesial temporal sclerosis. Epilepsy Res 2012;102:86–93.

118 Schmitz B: Depression and mania in patients with epilepsy. Epilepsia 2005;46(suppl 4):45–49.

119 Behrens E, Schramm J, Zentner J, Konig R: Surgical and neurological complications in a series of 708 epilepsy surgery procedures. Neurosurgery 1997; 41:1–9, discussion 9–10.

120 Elsharkawy AE, Alabbasi AH, Pannek H, Oppel F, Schulz R, Hoppe M, Hamad AP, Nayel M, Issa A, Ebner A: Long-term outcome after temporal lobe epilepsy surgery in 434 consecutive adult patients. J Neurosurg 2009;110:1135–1146.

121 Wieshmann UC, Larkin D, Varma T, Eldridge P: Predictors of outcome after temporal lobectomy for refractory temporal lobe epilepsy. Acta Neurol Scand 2008;118:306–312.

122 Acar G, Acar F, Miller J, Spencer DC, Burchiel KJ: Seizure outcome following transcortical selective amygdalohippocampectomy in mesial temporal lobe epilepsy. Stereotact Funct Neurosurg 2008;86:314–319.

123 Wieser HG, Ortega M, Friedman A, Yonekawa Y: Long-term seizure outcomes following amygdalohippocampectomy. J Neurosurg 2003;98:751–763.

124 Engel J, Van Ness PC, Rasmussen TB, Ojemann LM: Surgical Treatment of the Epilepsies. New York, Raven Press, 1993.

125 Wieser HG, Blume WT, Fish D, Goldensohn E, Hufnagel A, King D, Sperling MR, Luders H, Pedley TA: ILAE Commission Report. Proposal for a new classification of outcome with respect to epileptic seizures following epilepsy surgery. Epilepsia 2001;42:282–286.

126 Elliott RE, Bollo RJ, Berliner JL, Silverberg A, Carlson C, Geller EB, Barr WB, Devinsky O, Doyle WK: Anterior temporal lobectomy with amygdalohippocampectomy for mesial temporal sclerosis: predictors of long-term seizure control. J Neurosurg 2013;119:261–272.

127 Tonini C, Beghi E, Berg AT, Bogliun G, Giordano L, Newton RW, Tetto A, Vitelli E, Vitezic D, Wiebe S: Predictors of epilepsy surgery outcome: a meta-analysis. Epilepsy Res 2004;62:75–87.

128 Yang XL, Lu QC, Xu JW, Wang GS, Liu Q: Predictors of outcome in the surgical treatment for epilepsy. Chin Med J (Engl) 2011;124:4166–4171.

129 Jeong SW, Lee SK, Kim KK, Kim H, Kim JY, Chung CK: Prognostic factors in anterior temporal lobe resections for mesial temporal lobe epilepsy: multivariate analysis. Epilepsia 1999;40:1735–1739.

130 Mueller CA, Scorzin J, von Lehe M, Fimmers R, Helmstaedter C, Zentner J, Lehmann TN, Meencke HJ, Schulze-Bonhage A, Schramm J: Seizure outcome 1 year after temporal lobe epilepsy: an analysis of MR volumetric and clinical parameters. Acta Neurochir (Wien) 2012;154:1327–1336.

131 Smyth MD, Limbrick DDJ, Ojemann JG, Zempel J, Robinson S, O'Brien DF, Saneto RP, Goyal M, Appleton RE, Mangano FT, Park TS: Outcome following surgery for temporal lobe epilepsy with hippocampal involvement in preadolescent children: emphasis on mesial temporal sclerosis. J Neurosurg 2007;106:205–210.

132 Lee TM, Yip JT, Jones-Gotman M: Memory deficits after resection from left or right anterior temporal lobe in humans: a meta-analytic review. Epilepsia 2002;43:283–291.

133 Helmstaedter CA: Prediction of memory reserve capacity. Adv Neurol 1999;81:271–279.

134 Clusmann H, Schramm J, Kral T, Helmstaedter C, Ostertun B, Fimmers R, Haun D, Elger CE: Prognostic factors and outcome after different types of resection for temporal lobe epilepsy. J Neurosurg 2002;97:1131–1141.

135 Pauli E, Pickel S, Schulemann H, Buchfelder M, Stefan H: Neuropsychologic findings depending on the type of the resection in temporal lobe epilepsy. Adv Neurol 1999;81:371–377.

136 Wendling AS, Hirsch E, Wisniewski I, Davanture C, Ofer I, Zentner J, Bilic S, Scholly J, Staack AM, Valenti MP, Schulze-Bonhage A, Kehrli P, Steinhoff BJ: Selective amygdalohippocampectomy versus standard temporal lobectomy in patients with mesial temporal lobe epilepsy and unilateral hippocampal sclerosis. Epilepsy Res 2013;104:94–104.

137 Devinsky O, Barr WB, Vickrey BG, Berg AT, Bazil CW, Pacia SV, Langfitt JT, Walczak TS, Sperling MR, Shinnar S, Spencer SS: Changes in depression and anxiety after resective surgery for epilepsy. Neurology 2005;65:1744–1749.

138 Wilson SJ, Wrench JM, McIntosh AM, Bladin PF, Berkovic SF: Profiles of psychosocial outcome after epilepsy surgery: the role of personality. Epilepsia 2010;51:1133–1138.

139 Barbaro NM, Quigg M, Broshek DK, Ward MM, Lamborn KR, Laxer KD, Larson DA, Dillon W, Verhey L, Garcia P, Steiner L, Heck C, Kondziolka D, Beach R, Olivero W, Witt TC, Salanova V, Goodman R: A multicenter, prospective pilot study of gamma knife radiosurgery for mesial temporal lobe epilepsy: seizure response, adverse events, and verbal memory. Ann Neurol 2009;65:167–175.

140 Regis J, Rey M, Bartolomei F, Vladyka V, Liscak R, Schrottner O, Pendl G: Gamma knife surgery in mesial temporal lobe epilepsy: a prospective multicenter study. Epilepsia 2004;45:504–515.

141 Malikova H, Kramska L, Liscak R, Vojtech Z, Prochazka T, Mareckova I, Lukavsky J, Druga R: Stereotactic radiofrequency amygdalohippocampectomy for the treatment of temporal lobe epilepsy: do good neuropsychological and seizure outcomes correlate with hippocampal volume reduction? Epilepsy Res 2012;102:34–44.

142 Bartolomei F, Hayashi M, Tamura M, Rey M, Fischer C, Chauvel P, Regis J: Long-term efficacy of gamma knife radiosurgery in mesial temporal lobe epilepsy. Neurology 2008;70:1658–1663.

143 Finet P, Rooijakkers H, Godfraind C, Raftopoulos C: Delayed compressive angiomatous degeneration in a case of mesial temporal lobe epilepsy treated by gamma knife radiosurgery: case report. Neurosurgery 2010;67:218–220, discussion 220.

144 Kawamura T, Onishi H, Kohda Y, Hirose G: Serious adverse effects of gamma knife radiosurgery for mesial temporal lobe epilepsy. Neurol Med Chir (Tokyo) 2012;52:892–898.

145 Liang S, Liu T, Li A, Zhao M, Yu X, Qh O: Long-term follow up of very low-dose LINAC based stereotactic radiotherapy in temporal lobe epilepsy. Epilepsy Res 2010;90:60–67.

146 Vale FL, Bozorg AM, Schoenberg MR, Wong K, Witt TC: Long-term radiosurgery effects in the treatment of temporal lobe epilepsy. J Neurosurg 2012;117:962–969.

147 Velasco M, Velasco F, Velasco AL, Boleaga B, Jimenez F, Brito F, Marquez I: Subacute electrical stimulation of the hippocampus blocks intractable temporal lobe seizures and paroxysmal EEG activities. Epilepsia 2000;41:158–169.

148 Velasco AL, Velasco F, Velasco M, Trejo D, Castro G, Carrillo-Ruiz JD: Electrical stimulation of the hippocampal epileptic foci for seizure control: a double-blind, long-term follow-up study. Epilepsia 2007;48:1895–1903.

149 Velasco AL, Velasco F, Velasco M, Jimenez F, Carrillo-Ruiz JD, Castro G: The role of neuromodulation of the hippocampus in the treatment of intractable complex partial seizures of the temporal lobe. Acta Neurochir Suppl 2007;97:329–332.

150 Tellez-Zenteno JF, McLachlan RS, Parrent A, Kubu CS, Wiebe S: Hippocampal electrical stimulation in mesial temporal lobe epilepsy. Neurology 2006;66: 1490–1494.

151 Vonck K, Boon P, Achten E, De Reuck J, Caemaert J: Long-term amygdalohippocampal stimulation for refractory temporal lobe epilepsy. Ann Neurol 2002;52:556–565.

Dr. Anastasios Chatzikonstantinou
Department of Neurology, UniversitätsMedizin Mannheim
Theodor-Kutzer-Ufer 1-3
DE–68167 Mannheim (Germany)
E-Mail chatziko@neuro.ma.uni-heidelberg.de

Chatzikonstantinou

Szabo K, Hennerici MG (eds): The Hippocampus in Clinical Neuroscience.
Front Neurol Neurosci. Basel, Karger, 2014, vol 34, pp 143–149 (DOI: 10.1159/000356431)

Transient Global Amnesia

Kristina Szabo

Department of Neurology, UniversitätsMedizin Mannheim, University of Heidelberg, Mannheim, Germany

Abstract

Transient global amnesia (TGA) is a sudden and severe anterograde memory disturbance accompanied by various degrees of retrograde amnesia and sometimes executive dysfunction. TGA affects elderly individuals and men and women equally. During the episode, patients cannot recall novel episodic information and therefore repeatedly ask the same questions. They are not fully oriented to space and time. Diagnostic criteria first established in 1985, and elaborated in 1990, demand that there is no clouding of consciousness, other impairments of cognition, or a history of epilepsy or head trauma. An episode of TGA resolves within 24 h leaving a memory gap for the length of the attack. While in rare cases TGA might happen repeatedly, it mostly occurs as a single attack. TGA is considered a benign disorder as memory deficits resolve completely and do not lead to long-term sequelae. In up to 90% of reported TGA cases, a precipitating event – mainly described as physical or emotional stress – is present. The cause of TGA has been a matter of long-standing debate among researchers. In search of an answer, several possible causes (ischemia, migraine, epileptic seizures, or, more recently, a disturbance of venous hemodynamics) have been hypothesized. However, to date there is no scientific proof of any of these mechanisms. By using diffusion-weighted MRI 24–48 h after a TGA episode, small dot-like lesions have been detected in the hippocampus. This has led to the implication that the selective vulnerability of CA1 neurons to metabolic stress might play a role in the pathophysiology of TGA.

Historical Background

Transient global amnesia (TGA) is one of the most fascinating disorders in clinical neurology, and is characterized by a sudden attack of mainly anterograde amnesia accompanied by typical behavioral changes – both resolving within 24 h. According to Haas [1], the first description of such an attack was published by Hauge [2] in 1954 describing amnesia as a complication occurring in 3 patients after vertebral angiography. In a more recent historical note, Pearce and Bogousslavsky [3] claim, that the first report of a TGA-like attack might even date back to the year 1909, when Benon [4] described an 'ictus amnésique' with a sudden onset of retro- and anterograde amnesia of organic cause. At the time, Benon made the point to differentiate this entity from hysterical disturbances – considered to be one of the most common causes of memory impairment in the 19th century. In 1956, Bender [5] described a disorder in 12 elderly patients he termed 'syndrome of isolated episode of confusion with amnesia' with the inability to form new memories and repeatedly asking the same questions. He stressed in his observation that these were single episodes without recurrence. In the same year, Guyotat and Courjon [6] reported 16 cases of 'les ictus amnésiques' with temporary memory disturbance without further neurological deficits.

The term 'transient global amnesia' was introduced by the neurologists Fisher and Adams in 1958 and 1964 [7, 8], when they described 17 patients with abrupt onset of mainly anterograde amnesia. They reported in great detail the typical clinical characteristics of TGA, in particular the feature of repeated questions from the patients concerning the ongoing situation. This is an excerpt from one of their cases concerning a 55-year-old physician whose symptoms started while he was seeing one of his longtime patients:

> He told his patient he was having a lapse of memory, asked her who she was and why she was there. He asked over and over again what day it was and why his secretary was not available (he had given permission for a vacation ten days before)...

Other typical findings in their series of patients included the abrupt onset, the lack of neurological symptoms, the gradual recovery, and the remaining amnestic gap. In the following years, numerous reports describing these typical characteristics followed. In 1985, Caplan was the first to propose the following four operational criteria for TGA published in the *Handbook of Clinical Neurology* [9]:

- Information about the beginning of the attack should be available from a capable observer who witnesses the onset.
- The patient should have been examined during the attack to be certain that other neurological symptoms and signs did not accompany the amnesia.
- There should be no important accompanying neurological signs.
- The memory loss should be transient.

He stressed the importance of diagnostic boundaries, stating 'This task is admittedly difficult in a disorder when the etiology is uncertain and pathological anatomy and pathophysiology cannot be verified by laboratory or radiographic investigations.'

In 1990, Hodges and Warlow [10] modified Caplan's definitions and established the clinical diagnostic criteria that are still in use today (table 1). They reported 153 cases with acute transient amnesia, of which 114 fulfilled these criteria and had an excellent outcome. The group of 39 patients who did not meet these criteria had a significantly worse prognosis with a high incidence of major vascular events.

Demographic Features

The incidence of TGA is estimated as at least 3–10/100,000 per year and affects men and women equally [11–14]. Approximately 75% of TGA patients are between 50 and 80 years of age (mean: 60.3), and in most cases TGA occurs once in a lifetime [9, 14].

Table 1. Diagnostic criteria for TGA according to Hodges and Warlow [10]

1.	Attacks must be witnessed and information available from a capable observer who was present for most of the attack
2.	There must be a clear-cut anterograde amnesia during the attack
3.	Clouding of consciousness and loss of personal identity must be absent, and the cognitive impairment limited to amnesia (i.e. no aphasia, apraxia, etc.)
4.	There should be no accompanying focal neurological symptoms during the attack and no significant neurological signs afterwards
5.	Epileptic features must be absent
6.	Attacks must resolve within 24 h
7.	Patients with recent head injury or active epilepsy (i.e. remaining on medication or one seizure in the past 2 years) are excluded

In an estimated 6–10% of patients, however, TGA might occur repeatedly [14, 15]. Intervals between these episodes vary between months and years.

Certain aspects of personality have been suggested to be more common in TGA patients. In 1997, Inzitari et al. [16] found phobic personality traits in 82% of 51 TGA patients. Depressive symptoms and psychiatric comorbidities have also been claimed to be more common in TGA [17, 18]. In their series of 142 patients, Quinette et al. [14] reported a high frequency of psychological and emotional instability, suggesting that TGA patients might be particularly vulnerable to psychological stress. Even as early as 1964, the presence of certain events occurring immediately before the attack – such as swimming in cold water, taking hot showers, pain, and sexual intercourse – was described [8]. As analyzed more recently, in up to 90% (32–89.1%) of reported TGA cases, a precipitating event – mainly described as physical, emotional, or behavioral stress – has been reported [14]. In addition to those mentioned above, other typical events include stressful medical examinations, arguments, funerals, exhausting physical work, and celebrations [14, 19]. Besides events immediately before the attack, remote factors preceding TGA by days or weeks, e.g. anxiety, exhaustion, or financial worries, have also been described [14].

Clinical Presentation

TGA is characterized by a sudden attack of severe disturbance of anterograde episodic long-term memory, i.e. patients have difficulty in learning and subsequently recalling novel episodic information [20, 21]. In many but not all patients, a partial or 'patchy' impairment of retrograde episodic long-term memory is also present: patients have difficulty recalling episodic information that was learned (hours, days, months, or even years) before the onset of the amnestic attack [22]. Other cognitive functions such as short-term memory, semantic memory, or implicit and procedural memory are not affected at all [20, 22]. Recently, a significant reduction of executive function including working-memory processes during episodes of TGA has been demonstrated [22].

Typical TGA patients are slightly worried but not confused, and they repeatedly ask the same questions concerning their present whereabouts and situation ('How did I get here?', 'What am I doing here?'). They are cooperative, alert, and fully oriented to person, but not accurately to time and place, and they do not remember any novel information, e.g. the treating physician or why they were brought to hospital. While the lack of additional neurological symptoms is mandatory for the diagnosis of TGA, there are a number of associated symptoms reported in the literature, such as headache, nausea, emesis, dizziness, chills/flushes, fear of dying, emotionalism, etc. [14, 23]. The exact duration of a TGA episode is often difficult to determine as recovery is mostly gradual. Once TGA has ended, the patient is able to recall hospital events (e.g. names of doctors) and report the reason for the hospital stay. As defined in the clinical criteria, TGA must resolve within 24 h; however, the typical duration reported in studies is in general shorter, estimated to be between 4 and 6 h [11, 14]. Almost all reported cases have a permanent memory gap for the duration of the attack [9]. Many (but not all) studies have shown complete recovery of memory functioning several months after an episode of TGA [24–29]. However, the recovery of TGA-induced memory deficits has been shown to be somewhat delayed and gradual, as slightly poorer performance in the affected cognitive domains seems to be also present in the postacute phase of the disorder [22, 30, 31].

Etiological Considerations

The cause of TGA has been a matter of long-standing debate among researchers. Several groups have suggested that the pathophysiological mechanisms leading to the memory disturbance may be similar to those of cerebral ischemia, epilepsy, or migraine [32, 33]. However, there is no definitive evidence supporting any of these mechanisms. In addition, there is no evidence for an increased rate or intensity of cerebrovascular risk factors, microangiopathy, or ischemic strokes in TGA patients [34, 35]. More recently, a disturbance of venous hemodynamics has been hypothesized, but again without any scientific proof for such an underlying mechanism [36]. Due to the nature of the cognitive impairment during TGA, a transient dysfunction of the medial temporal lobes, especially of the hippocampus, has been repeatedly postulated [37]. Dysfunction of the prefrontal cortex has also been suspected to be involved in the development of a TGA episode [38]. Neuroimaging studies in single patients or small case series using PET or SPECT have shown alterations of perfusion or metabolism during the acute or postacute phase of TGA in the thalamus, amygdala, medial temporal lobes, and prefrontal cortex [38, 39].

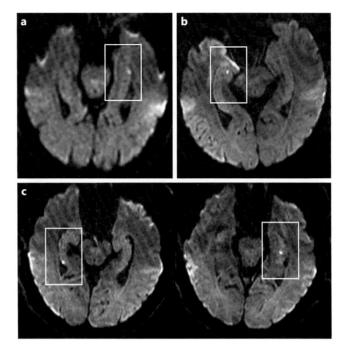

Fig. 1. Diffusion-weighted MRI parallel to the long axis of the hippocampus shows a typical hyperintense dot-like lesion in the left (**a**) or right (**b**) hippocampus. In some patients, multiple lesions are found involving the hippocampus bilaterally (**c**).

In 1999, Gass et al. [40] examined patients with acute TGA using MRI and found no signs of hyperintensity on diffusion-weighted MRI that would imply the regional decrease of water mobility or acute T2 signal changes. The lack of such findings suggested that mechanisms other than ischemic infarction cause TGA. Extending this research in a follow-up study, the group used a modified study design to investigate TGA patients that included serial diffusion-weighted MRI measurements performed from the day of symptom onset through days 1 and 2 [41]. As a result, they were able to demonstrate that more than 80% of patients developed a small, point-shaped uni- or bilateral diffusion-weighted MRI lesion in the lateral aspect of the hippocampal formation that became detectable 48 h after symptom onset (fig. 1). These results have been confirmed by other groups since, and while this finding actually linked the disorder to the CA1 subfield of the hippocampus anatomically, the exact etiology of these small lesions still remains uncertain [24].

Another hypothesis postulates that the disorder is caused by the stress-related transient inhibition of memory formation in the hippocampus. Activation of the hypothalamus-pituitary-adrenal axis during accidental or experimentally induced stress is known to lead to an elevation of stress hormone levels. High glucocorticoid levels in turn have been shown to increase neuronal vulnerability in the hippocampus, induce a decrease in regional cerebral blood flow in the mesial temporal lobe, and have a negative effect on cognition and memory [42]. To test this assumption, an ongoing study is examining the effect of experimental exposure to stress on stress hormone levels and hippocampal activation patterns using functional MRI in TGA patients [43].

References

1   Haas DC: Transient global amnesia after cerebral angiography. Arch Neurol 1983;40:258–259.
2   Hauge T: Catheter vertebral angiography. Acta Radiol Suppl 1954;109:1–219.
3   Pearce JM, Bogousslavsky J: 'Les ictus amnesiques' and transient global amnesia. Eur Neurol 2009;62:188–192.
4   Benon R: Les ictus amnésiques dans les démences 'organiques'. Ann Méd Psychol 1909;67:207–219.
5   Bender M: Syndrome of isolated episode of confusion with amnesia. J Hillside Hosp 1956;5:212–215.
6   Guyotat MM, Courjon J: Les ictus amnésiques. J Med Lyon 1956;37:697–701.
7   Fisher CM, Adams RD: Transient global amnesia. Trans Am Neurol Assoc 1958;83:143–146.
8   Fisher CM, Adams RD: Transient global amnesia. Acta Neurol Scand Suppl 1964;40(suppl 9):1–83.
9   Caplan LR: Transient global amnesia; in Vinken PJ, Bruyn GW, Klawans HL (eds): Handbook of Clinical Neurology. Amsterdam, Elsevier, 1985, vol 45, pp 205–218.
10 Hodges JR, Warlow CP: The aetiology of transient global amnesia. A case-control study of 114 cases with prospective follow-up. Brain 1990;113:639–657.
11 Zeman AZ, Hodges JR: Transient global amnesia. Br J Hosp Med 1997;58:257–260.
12 Berli R, Hutter A, Waespe W, Bachli EB: Transient global amnesia – not so rare after all. Swiss Med Wkly 2009;139:288–292.
13 Miller JW, Petersen RC, Metter EJ, Millikan CH, Yanagihara T: Transient global amnesia: clinical characteristics and prognosis. Neurology 1987;37:733–737.
14 Quinette P, Guillery-Girard B, Dayan J, de la Sayette V, Marquis S, Viader F, Desgranges B, Eustache F: What does transient global amnesia really mean? Review of the literature and thorough study of 142 cases. Brain 2006;129:1640–1658.
15 Agosti C, Akkawi NM, Borroni B, Padovani A: Recurrency in transient global amnesia: a retrospective study. Eur J Neurol 2006;13:986–989.
16 Inzitari D, Pantoni L, Lamassa M, Pallanti S, Pracucci G, Marini P: Emotional arousal and phobia in transient global amnesia. Arch Neurol 1997;54:866–873.
17 Pantoni L, Bertini E, Lamassa M, Pracucci G, Inzitari D: Clinical features, risk factors, and prognosis in transient global amnesia: a follow-up study. Eur J Neurol 2005;12:350–356.
18 Neri M, Andermarcher E, De Vreese LP, Rubichi S, Sacchet C, Cipolli C: Transient global amnesia: memory and metamemory. Aging 1995;7:423–429.
19 Markowitsch HJ: Transient global amnesia. Neurosci Biobehav Rev 1983;7:35–43.
20 Jager T, Szabo K, Griebe M, Bazner H, Moller J, Hennerici MG: Selective disruption of hippocampus-mediated recognition memory processes after episodes of transient global amnesia. Neuropsychologia 2009;47:70–76.
21 Mazzucchi A, Parma M: Neuropsychological testing of transient global amnesia during attack and during follow-up; in Markowitsch HJ (ed): Transient Global Amnesia and Related Disorders. Toronto, Hogrefe & Huber, 1990, pp 152–167.
22 Jager T, Bazner H, Kliegel M, Szabo K, Hennerici MG: The transience and nature of cognitive impairments in transient global amnesia: a meta-analysis. J Clin Exp Neuropsychol 2009;31:8–19.
23 Hodges JR, Oxbury SM: Persistent memory impairment following transient global amnesia. J Clin Exp Neuropsychol 1990;12:904–920.
24 Bartsch T, Alfke K, Stingele R, Rohr A, Freitag-Wolf S, Jansen O, Deuschl G: Selective affection of hippocampal CA-1 neurons in patients with transient global amnesia without long-term sequelae. Brain 2006;129:2874–2884.
25 Faglioni P, Scarpa M, Colombo A, Botti C, Grisanti A: A model-based study of learning and memory following transient global amnesia attacks. Cortex 1992;28:9–22.
26 Kritchevsky M, Squire LR: Transient global amnesia: evidence for extensive, temporally graded retrograde amnesia. Neurology 1989;39:213–218.
27 Kritchevsky M, Squire LR, Zouzounis JA: Transient global amnesia: characterization of anterograde and retrograde amnesia. Neurology 1988;38:213–219.
28 Quinette P, Guillery B, Desgranges B, de la Sayette V, Viader F, Eustache F: Working memory and executive functions in transient global amnesia. Brain 2003;126:1917–1934.
29 Uttner I, Weber S, Freund W, Schmitz B, Ramspott M, Huber R: Transient global amnesia – full recovery without persistent cognitive impairment. Eur Neurol 2007;58:146–151.
30 Hodges JR, Ward CD: Observations during transient global amnesia. A behavioural and neuropsychological study of five cases. Brain 1989;112:595–620.
31 Kessler J, Markowitsch HJ, Rudolf J, Heiss WD: Continuing cognitive impairment after isolated transient global amnesia. Int J Neurosci 2001;106:159–168.
32 Frederiks JA: Transient global amnesia. Clin Neurol Neurosurg 1993;95:265–283.
33 Tong DC, Grossman M: What causes transient global amnesia? New insights from DWI. Neurology 2004;62:2154–2155.

34 Enzinger C, Thimary F, Kapeller P, Ropele S, Schmidt R, Ebner F, Fazekas F: Transient global amnesia: diffusion-weighted imaging lesions and cerebrovascular disease. Stroke 2008;39:2219–2225.

35 Zorzon M, Antonutti L, Mase G, Biasutti E, Vitrani B, Cazzato G: Transient global amnesia and transient ischemic attack. Natural history, vascular risk factors, and associated conditions. Stroke 1995;26:1536–1542.

36 Baracchini C, Tonello S, Farina F, Viaro F, Atzori M, Ballotta E, Manara R: Jugular veins in transient global amnesia: innocent bystanders. Stroke 2012;43:2289–2292.

37 Bartsch T, Deuschl G: Transient global amnesia: functional anatomy and clinical implications. Lancet Neurol 2010;9:205–214.

38 Eustache F, Desgranges B, Petit-Taboué MC, de la Sayette V, Piot V, Sablé C, Marchal G, Baron JC: Transient global amnesia: implicit/explicit memory dissociation and PET assessment of brain perfusion and oxygen metabolism in the acute stage. J Neurol Neurosurg Psychiatry 1997;63:357–367.

39 Baron JC, Petit-Taboue MC, Le Doze F, Desgranges B, Ravenel N, Marchal G: Right frontal cortex hypometabolism in transient global amnesia. A PET study. Brain 1994;117:545–552.

40 Gass A, Gaa J, Hirsch J, Schwartz A, Hennerici MG: Lack of evidence of acute ischemic tissue change in transient global amnesia on single-shot echo-planar diffusion-weighted MRI. Stroke 1999;30:2070–2072.

41 Sedlaczek O, Hirsch JG, Grips E, Peters CN, Gass A, Wohrle J, Hennerici M: Detection of delayed focal MR changes in the lateral hippocampus in transient global amnesia. Neurology 2004;62:2165–2170.

42 Lupien SJ, Lepage M: Stress, memory, and the hippocampus: can't live with it, can't live without it. Behav Brain Res 2001;127:137–158.

43 Griebe M, Hennerici MG, Szabo K: Letter by Griebe et al regarding article. Jugular veins in transient global amnesia: innocent bystanders. Stroke 2012;43:e165, author reply e166.

Prof. Dr. Kristina Szabo
Department of Neurology, UniversitätsMedizin Mannheim
Theodor-Kutzer-Ufer 1-3
DE–68167 Mannheim (Germany)
E-Mail szabo@neuro.ma.uni-heidelberg.de

Szabo K, Hennerici MG (eds): The Hippocampus in Clinical Neuroscience.
Front Neurol Neurosci. Basel, Karger, 2014, vol 34, pp 150–156 (DOI: 10.1159/000356438)

Hippocampal Stroke

Kristina Szabo

Department of Neurology, UniversitätsMedizin Mannheim, University of Heidelberg, Mannheim, Germany

Abstract

The first to link disturbance of memory and lesions of the medial temporal lobe was the Russian neurologist von Bechterew, who in 1989 presented the brain of a 60-year-old man who had suffered from severe amnesia. Autopsy showed bilateral damage of the medial temporal lobe. Several following postmortem case studies confirmed the association between permanent amnesia and bitemporal stroke. Reports of transient memory deficits in unilateral stroke in combination with other neurological and neuropsychological deficits followed. With the advent of brain imaging, persistent or transient amnesia as the sole or primary manifestation of acute – mostly left-sided – hippocampal stroke was described. With the use of modern MRI techniques the identification of typical ischemic stroke lesion patterns affecting the hippocampus has become possible. Although overt cognitive deficits in unilateral hippocampal stroke seem to be rare, a careful neuropsychological examination might be necessary to detect resulting neuropsychological deficits including disturbances of verbal and nonverbal episodic long-term memory and spatial orientation.

© 2014 S. Karger AG, Basel

From basic neuroscience studies of histopathology, it is well known that cerebral ischemia may be classified as global (affecting the entire brain) or focal (affecting a specific region), with different patterns of spatial and temporal evolution and different histopathological correlates. In rats, the severity and duration of transient occlusion of all cerebral vessels has been shown to lead to delayed selective damage of hippocampal CA1 neurons while leaving other cell types in the hippocampus undamaged. This observation has led to the term 'selective vulnerability' and has been explained by the long-term effects of high levels of glutamate [1]. Other regions vulnerable to global cerebral ischemia include the thalamic nuclei, the basal ganglia, and the brainstem. Global cerebral ischemia in a clinical setting occurs in cardiac arrest or severe hypotension, and may lead to selective ischemic necrosis.

In contrast, focal cerebral ischemia – referred to as 'stroke' in clinical practice – is encountered when a cerebral arterial vessel is occluded by local atherosclerosis or embolism. The resulting final tissue infarction depends on the degree and duration of vessel occlusion and the patency of collaterals. In humans, the hippocampus, as part of the network of the limbic system is a particularly interesting anatomical structure because of its critical role in learning, memory, and emotional behavior in addition to it being affected by a variety of pathologies ranging from acute infection to neurodegeneration. Descriptions of acute ischemic stroke lesions affecting the hippocampus and its symptomatology, however, are rare. Much of the progress in the understanding of hippocampal pathologies has been made since the use of MRI, but there is little morphological information concerning hippocampal stroke.

Early Anatomical Studies of Hippocampal Stroke

In 1900, the neurologist and psychiatrist Wladimir von Bechterew [2] from St. Petersburg, Russia, described a patient with bilateral softening involving the uncus and Ammon's horn revealed on postmortem examination. He reported that the 60-year-old man had suffered from remarkable amnesia, false memories, and apathy since the age of 40. This is believed to be the first report linking memory deficit to the temporal lobe in humans.

In the second half of the 20th century, numerous reports established bilateral temporal lobe damage – of different etiology – as a cause of severe and persistent amnesia. In 1961, Victor et al. [3] published a postmortem study of a patient with permanent memory disturbance due to *bilateral* infarctions in the posterior cerebral stroke (PCA) territories. Van Buren and Borke [4] in 1972 reported histological findings in 2 patients with persistent severe memory loss and spatial disorientation. One of them had bilateral PCA strokes due to a large aneurysm of the basilar artery; in the other case, successive strokes in both hemispheres involving temporal lobe structures had led to a severe spatial disorientation with memory difficulty and a restricted visual field.

Several postmortem cases also reported transient amnesia occurring in *unilateral* PCA stroke. In 1966, Geschwind and Fusillo [5] reported the case of a patient with alexia without agraphia and a transient disturbance of memory. This patient had unilateral PCA infarction involving the occipital lobe, hippocampus, and thalamus. A similar case was that of a 72-year-old man with a circumscribed ischemic stroke in the left PCA territory with involvement of the lateral geniculate body, hippocampus, and lateral dorsal nucleus as well as the pulvinar of the thalamus reported by Mohr et al. [6]. He had suffered sudden onset of partial right homonymous hemianopia with memory and color deficits. The memory disturbance was characterized as 'retro- and anterograde amnesia for the events surrounding the hospital admission, faulty retention of verbal material, impaired retention of a form discrimination test, and an amnestic dysnomia.' In their summary, the authors state, that '...a unilateral left hippo-campal infarct appears to be the most circumscribed lesion yet reported with memo-ry deficits.' In 1974, Caplan and Hedley-Whyte [7] reported a postmortem case with cueing and memory dysfunction in alexia without agraphia in a 68-year-old woman with an extensive left PCA stroke of cardiac origin. The common feature in all of these cases was the unilateral involvement of the dominant hippocampus and a temporary amnestic syndrome lasting several weeks to months.

Imaging Studies in Hippocampal Stroke

In 1974, Benson et al. [8] published a series of 10 patients in whom memory distur-bance was associated with either unilateral or bilateral visual field defects in PCA ter-ritory strokes (6 bilateral, 4 unilateral left sided) on radionuclide brain scans. In their report, they coined the term 'amnesic stroke'. In 1993, Ott and Saver [9] described the imaging (CT/MRI) and clinical findings in 6 patients with persistent or transient am-nesia as the sole or primary manifestation of acute – left-sided – ischemic or hemor-rhagic stroke. Five of these patients had PCA territory lesions involving the hippo-campus, and in 1 patient the anterior thalamus was affected. Reviewing the literature, the authors concluded that in 85% of the published cases, amnesia was caused by left-sided hippocampal stroke. However, they argued that this might be caused by selec-tion bias as left-hippocampal verbal memory deficits may be more evident than vi-sual memory disturbances in right hippocampal lesions. In the following years, the term 'amnesic stroke' was used to describe cases of acute amnesia of different vascular origins: PCA stroke, thalamic artery stroke, and anterior choroidal artery stroke. In 1997, an MRI study by Takahashi et al. [10] evaluated hippocampal involvement in PCA stroke in 14 patients. In 57% with either left or bilateral hippocampal stroke, an amnestic syndrome was reported. In this retrospective study, conventional T2-weight-ed sequences were analyzed, but no neuropsychological data was available.

Our group examined the MR morphological findings of diffusion-weighted MRI in hippocampal stroke and attempted to detect clinical and neuropsychological changes in acute hippocampal stroke patients [11]. We studied 57 patients consecu-tively admitted to the stroke unit of our hospital with acute ischemic stroke in the posterior circulation and diffusion-weighted MRI proven involvement of the hippo-campus (n = 60 affected hippocampi). In most patients, the acute presenting clinical symptoms arose from functional loss of posterior circulation lesions outside the hip-pocampus: visual field defects, sensorimotor hemiparesis, and hemisensory deficits (fig. 1).

Apparent clinical acute amnestic syndromes were present in only 19.3% of the pa-tients, including those with bilateral hippocampal stroke. We were able to identify four phenotypical lesion patterns in hippocampal stroke that usually occurs as part of multifocal PCA ischemia. Figure 2 shows nearly the complete hippocampus with ex-

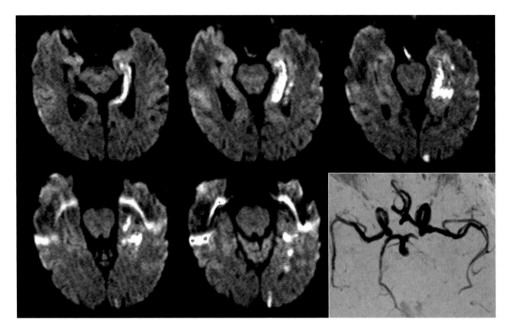

Fig. 1. Acute stroke MRI of a 68-year-old man who has been brought to the ER by his relatives. They reported that he had complained about visual disturbance and had seemed confused: diffusion-weighted MRI shows hyperintense ischemic lesions affecting the lateral hippocampus and the occipital lobe on the left. MRA indicates P2-segment stenosis/occlusion of the left PCA.

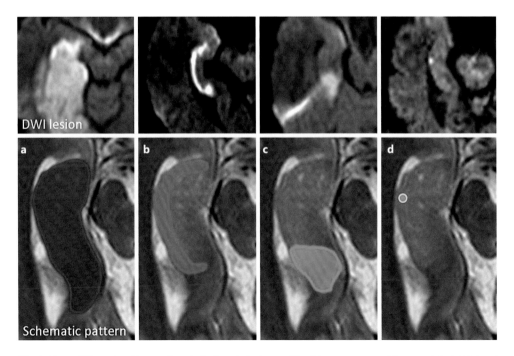

Fig. 2. Four different patterns of acute ischemic lesions of the hippocampus with complete (**a**), lateral (**b**), or dorsal (**c**) hippocampal lesions, and small circumscribed lesions in the lateral hippocampus (**d**).

Table 1. Neuropsychological tests

Test	Test procedure	Normative data
Rivermead Behavioural Memory Test	Memorize a short story and recall it immediately and after a delay of 20 min	Normative sample of German controls [15]
Auditory Verbal Learning Test	1. Memorize and recall a list of 15 words across five learning trials 2. Learn and recall a second list of 15 words in a single trial 3. Recall the words of the first list 4. After a delay of 30 min, recall the words of the first list 5. Recognize the 15 words among 76 written words	German version of the Auditory Verbal Learning Test [15]
Rey-Osterrieth Complex Figure Test	Copy a complex figure and recall it once after 3 min and once after 30 min	Meta-analysis [16]

tensive extrahippocampal involvement (complete or subtotal PCA stroke; fig. 2a), lesions confined to the lateral aspect of the hippocampus along the complete length of the hippocampal body and tail (fig. 2b), partial lesions in the dorsal part of the hippocampal body (fig. 2c), and small dot-like lesions in the lateral border of the hippocampus (fig. 2d). In all patients with hippocampal stroke, multiple acute ischemic lesions were found involving extrahippocampal tissue in the PCA territory. We compared neuropsychological test performance of right versus left hippocampal stroke in the last 20 patients of this series according to a protocol shown in table 1. We found significant long-term memory deficits, involving verbal episodic long-term memory in patients with left hippocampal stroke and nonverbal episodic long-term memory in patients with right hippocampal stroke, confirming the assumption of Ott and Saver [9] (fig. 3, 4).

Besides verbal and visual memory function, the hippocampus is believed to play a role in spatial navigation processing [12]. Maguire et al. [12] showed that London taxi drivers – who undergo extensive navigation training – have larger posterior hippocampal volumes than bus drivers. Interestingly, in a recent case report of a 70-year-old patient, right posterior hippocampal stroke was assumed to be the cause of acute loss of spatial navigational skills, a mild dysexecutive syndrome, and disturbance of visuospatial memory. The patient, a former hospital employee, decided to go to the ER because of unsteady gait, but drove aimlessly without finding the way to the place where he had worked for 20 years [13].

Although overt cognitive deficits in unilateral hippocampal stroke are rare, a careful neuropsychological examination might be necessary to detect resulting neuropsychological deficits. A recent study has suggested that stroke lesions in the hippocam-

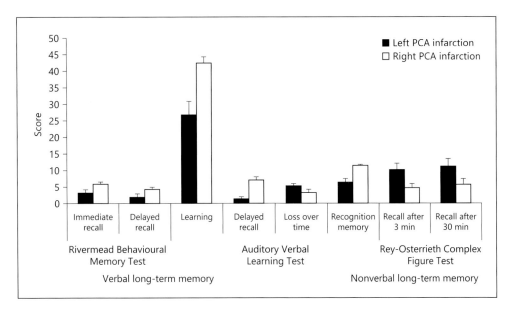

Fig. 3. Results of neuropsychological testing in means (plus standard errors) for performance of patients with left vs. right posterior cerebral artery infarction and corresponding hippocampal lesions in three tests of episodic long-term memory. From [11].

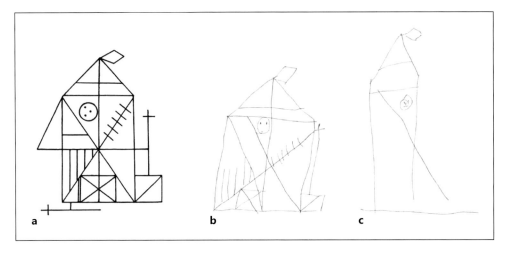

Fig. 4. Rey-Osterrieth Complex Figure Test (**a**) in a patient with right hippocampal stroke. The 57-year-old man was asked to copy the figure (**b**), then asked to redraw the figure from memory 30 min later (**c**).

pus may become relevant in the presence of a second pathology like Alzheimer dementia. The combination of the two pathologies may lead to the unmasking and decompensation of a fragile compensated functional state and may thereby be important in the physiopathology of mixed vascular dementia and Alzheimer's disease [14].

References

1 Benveniste H, Jorgensen MB, Sandberg M, Christensen T, Hagberg H, Diemer NH: Ischemic damage in hippocampal CA1 is dependent on glutamate release and intact innervation from CA3. J Cereb Blood Flow Metab 1989;9:629–639.

2 Bechterew W: Demonstration eines Gehirns mit Zerstörung der vorderen und inneren Teile der Hirnrinde beider Schläfenlappen. Neurol Zentralbl 1900;19:990–991.

3 Victor M, Angevine JB, Mancall EL, Fisher CM: Memory loss with lesions of hippocampal formation. Report of a case with some remarks on the anatomical basis of memory. Arch Neurol 1961;5:244–263.

4 Van Buren JM, Borke RC: The mesial temporal substratum of memory. Anatomical studies in three individuals. Brain 1972;95:599–632.

5 Geschwind N, Fusillo M: Color-naming defects in association with alexia. Arch Neurol 1966;15:137–146.

6 Mohr JP, Leicester J, Stoddard LT, Sidman M: Right hemianopia with memory and color deficits in circumscribed left posterior cerebral artery territory infarction. Neurology 1971;21:1104–1113.

7 Caplan LR, Hedley-Whyte T: Cuing and memory dysfunction in alexia without agraphia. A case report. Brain 1974;97:251–262.

8 Benson DF, Marsden CD, Meadows JC: The amnesic syndrome of posterior cerebral artery occlusion. Acta Neurol Scand 1974;50:133–145.

9 Ott BR, Saver JL: Unilateral amnesic stroke. Six new cases and a review of the literature. Stroke 1993;24:1033–1042.

10 Takahashi S, Higano S, Kurihara N, Mugikura S, Sakamoto K, Nomura H, Ikeda H: Correlation of lesions in the hippocampal region noted on MR images with clinical features. Eur Radiol 1997;7:281–286.

11 Szabo K, Forster A, Jager T, Kern R, Griebe M, Hennerici MG, Gass A: Hippocampal lesion patterns in acute posterior cerebral artery stroke: clinical and MRI findings. Stroke 2009;40:2042–2045.

12 Maguire EA, Gadian DG, Johnsrude IS, Good CD, Ashburner J, Frackowiak RS, Frith CD: Navigation-related structural change in the hippocampi of taxi drivers. Proc Natl Acad Sci USA 2000;97:4398–4403.

13 Aradillas E, Libon DJ, Schwartzman RJ: Acute loss of spatial navigational skills in a case of a right posterior hippocampus stroke. J Neurol Sci 2011;308:144–146.

14 Del Ser T, Hachinski V, Merskey H, Munoz DG: Alzheimer's disease with and without cerebral infarcts. J Neurol Sci 2005;231:3–11.

15 Helmstaedter C, Lendt M, Lux S: VLMT (Verbaler Lern- und Merkfaehigkeitstest): Manual. Goettingen, Beltz Test GmbH, 2001.

16 Mitrushina M, Boone KB, Razani J, D'Elia LF: Handbook of Normative Data for Neuropsychological Assessment, ed 2. New York, Oxford University Press, 2005.

Prof. Dr. Kristina Szabo
Department of Neurology, UniversitätsMedizin Mannheim
Theodor-Kutzer-Ufer 1-3
DE–68167 Mannheim (Germany)
E-Mail szabo@neuro.ma.uni-heidelberg.de

Author Index

Subject Index

Place cell, memory-related activity
  patterns 28, 29
Positron emission tomography
  Alzheimer's disease 102, 104, 105
  epilepsy 130, 131
Posttraumatic stress disorder
  functional magnetic resonance imaging 87,
    92, 93
  memory function 114
  stress effects
    cortisol effects on memory 115, 116
    hypothalamic-pituitary-adrenal axis
      alterations 114
    neuroimaging 115
Presenelin, mutations and Alzheimer's disease
  susceptibility 98

Recognition Memory Test 64
Rey Auditory Verbal Learning Test 63, 64
Rey-Osterrieth Complex Figure Test 66, 154,
  155
Ribot, Theodule-Armand 3
Rivermead Behavioural Memory Test II 64,
  154

Schizophrenia
  gene expression regulation in
    monkeys 46–48
  pathology in humans 45, 46
  susceptibility genes 47
Sclerosis, see Hippocampal sclerosis
Seizure, see also Epilepsy
  astrocyte coverage, febrile seizure
    role 43–45
  diffusion-weighted imaging of
    hippocampus 80, 81
Serial Reaction Time Test 68
Sharp-wave ripple complex 29, 30
Single photon emission computed tomography,
  Alzheimer's disease 102, 103
Stress
  hypothalamic-pituitary-adrenal axis 109,
    110
  memory effects
    borderline personality disorder
      clinical features 116
      cortisol effects on memory 117
      hypothalamic-pituitary-adrenal axis
        alterations 116, 117
      neuroimaging 117
    major depressive disorder

cortisol effects on memory 113, 114
hypothalamic-pituitary-adrenal axis
  alterations 112
memory function 111, 112
neuroimaging 112, 113
posttraumatic stress disorder
  cortisol effects on memory 115, 116
  hypothalamic-pituitary-adrenal axis
    alterations 114
  memory function 114
  neuroimaging 115
prospects for study 118
stress hormones 110, 111
Stroke
  diffusion-weighted imaging of
    hippocampus in acute ischemic
    stroke 77, 78, 152, 153
  history of hippocampal stroke studies 151,
    152
  neuropsychological assessment of
    hippocampal stroke 154, 155
  overview 150, 151
Subcortical connections, hippocampus 14, 15
Subiculum
  cytoarchitecture 11
  development in monkeys 42

Tau, phosphorylation in Alzheimer's
  disease 97
Transient global amnesia
  clinical presentation 145, 146
  demographics 144, 145
  diagnostic criteria 145
  diffusion-weighted imaging of
    hippocampus 78–80, 147
  etiology 146, 147
  history of study 143, 144

Uncal apex 22

Vascular dementia, hippocampus changes 104,
  105
Vascularization, hippocampus
  arteries
    deep 24
    superficial 22–24
  veins 24
Visuospatial function, assessment 65–68

Wechsler Memory Scale-III 63, 65
Wisconsin Card Sorting Test 64